# ABC OF
# EYES

## Fourth Edition

To our parents
who taught us to help and teach others

# ABC OF EYES

Fourth Edition

**P T Khaw PhD FRCP FRCS FRCOphth FRCPath FIBiol FMedSci**
*Professor and Consultant Ophthalmic Surgeon*
*Moorfields Eye Hospital and Institute of Ophthalmology*
*University College London*

**P Shah BSc(Hons) MB ChB FRCOphth**
*Consultant Ophthalmic Surgeon*
*The Birmingham and Midland Eye Centre and Good Hope Hospital NHS Trust*

*and*

**A R Elkington CBE MA FRCS FRCOphth(Hon) FCS(SA) Ophth(Hon)**
*Emeritus Professor of Ophthalmology*
*University of Southampton*
*Formerly President, Royal College of Ophthalmologists (1994–1997)*

First edition 1988
Second edition 1994
Third edition 1999
Fourth edition 2004
8        2010
by BMJ Publishing Group Ltd, BMA House, Tavistock Square,
London WC1H 9JR

www.bmjbooks.com

**British Library Cataloguing in Publication Data**
A catalogue record for this book is available from the British Library

ISBN : 978 0 7279 1659 4

Typeset by Newgen Imaging Systems (P) Ltd., Chennai, India
Printed and bound in Spain by Graphycems, Navarra
The cover shows a computer-enhanced blue/grey iris of the eye.
With permission of David Parker/Science Photo Library

# Contents

# Acknowledgements

We would like to acknowledge the help we have received over the years from our general practitioner, medical student, and ophthalmological colleagues for their probing questions that have helped us crystallise our thoughts on many topics. We are grateful to Alan Lacey from the Department of Medical Illustration at Moorfields Eye Hospital for his superb artistry and the diagrams. We would also like to thank Peggy Khaw for her tremendous work on the many drafts of the book from its inception, and Jennifer Murray for her help with the 4th edition. In the past Jane Smith, Mary Evans, Mary Banks, Deborah Reece, Alex Stibbe, and currently Eleanor Lines and Sally Carter have also been very supportive, steering us through the pitfalls of publishing. We also thank Steve Tuft for his expert advice on the refractive surgery section and Marie Tsaloumas for the photographs of age-related macular degeneration. Jackie Martin (supported by the Royal London Society for the Blind), Barbara Norton, and Jennifer Rignold guided us through the services for the visually handicapped. We thank Pharmacia (now Pfizer) for permission to use their colour plates on cataract surgery (page 48), Guide Dogs for the Blind for the picture of the guide dog (page 43), and Simon Keightley of the DVLA for his advice on driving standards. We are grateful to many people and organisations for use of their photographs in Chapter 14. These include the International Resource Centre for the Prevention of Blindness at the International Centre for Eye Health, London School of Hygiene and Tropical Medicine, London; Sue Stevens; John DC Anderson; Pak Sang Lee; Murray McGavin; Hugh Taylor; the Christoffel-Blindenmission (CBM); and the World Health Organization (the photograph of corneal melt on page 83 is from their Primary Eye Care slide set). The map on page 83 showing areas affected by onchoceriasis is adapted from a slide from the Image Bureau. Most of the photographs are copyright of Professor Peng Khaw. Some photographs are copyright of Moorfields Eye Hospital NHS Trust. The photograph of postoperative glaucoma drainage bleb on page 85 is copyright of City Hospital NHS Trust, Birmingham. We would like to acknowledge the support of the Michael and Ilse Katz Foundation.

PTK
PS
ARE
2004

# ABC of Eyes CD Rom

## Features

**ABC of Eyes PDF eBook**
- Bookmarked and hyperlinked for instant access to all headings and topics
- Fully indexed and searchable text—just click the "Search Text" button

**Artwork slideshow**
- Every diagram and photograph from the book, organised by chapter
- Hover over a image thumbnail and the caption will appear in a pop-up window
- Click on the image thumbnail to view at full-screen size, then use the left and right cursor keys to view the previous or next figure

**PDA Edition sample chapter**
- A chapter from *ABC of Eyes*, adpted for use on handheld devices such as *Palm* and *Pocket PC*
- Click on the underlined text to view an image (or images) relevant to the text concerned
- Use Mobipocket Reader technology, compatible with all PDA devices and also available for Windows
- Follow the on-screen instructions on the relevant part of the CD Rom to install Mobipocket for your device
- Full title available in this format for purchase as a download from http://www.pda.bmjbooks.com

**BMJ Books catalogue**
- Instant access to BMJ Books full catalogue, including an order form

## Instructions for use

The CD Rom should start automatically upon insertion, on all Windows systems. The menu screen will appear and you can then navigate by clicking on the headings. If the CD Rom does not start automatically upon insertion, please browse using "Windows Explorer" and double-click the file "BMJ_Books.exe".

## Tips

To minimise the bookmarks pane so that you can zoom the page to full screen width, simply click on the "Bookmarks" tab on the left of your screen. The bookmarks can be accessed again at any time by simply clicking this tab again.
To search the text simply click on "Search Text", then type into the window provided. You can stop the search at any time by clicking "Stop Search", and can then navigate directly to a search result by double-clicking on the specific result in the Search pane. By clicking your left mouse button once on a page in the PDF ebook window, you "activate" the window. You can now scroll through pages uses the scroll-wheel on your mouse, or by using the cursor keys on your keyboard.

*Note*: the ABC of Eyes PDF eBook is for on-screen search and reference only and cannot be printed. A printable PDF version as well as the full PDA edition can be purchased from http://www.bmjbookshop.com

## Troubleshooting

If any problems are experienced with use of the CD Rom, we can give you access to all content* via the internet. Please send your CD Rom with proof of purchase to the following address, with a letter advising your email address and the problem you have encountered:

ABC of Eyes eBook access
BMJ Bookshop
BMA House
Tavistock Square
London
WC1H 9JR

*Unfortunately, due to technical limitations, this offer currently excludes the artwork slideshow

# 1 History and examination

## History

As in all clinical medicine, an accurate history and examination are essential for correct diagnosis and treatment. Most ocular conditions can be diagnosed with a good history and simple examination techniques. Conversely, the failure to take a history and perform a simple examination can lead to conditions being missed that pose a threat to sight, or even to life.

The history may give many clues to the diagnosis. Visual symptoms are particularly important.

The rate of onset of visual symptoms gives an indication of the cause. A sudden deterioration in vision tends to be vascular in origin, whereas a gradual onset suggests a cause such as cataract. The loss of visual field may be characteristic, such as the central field loss of macular degeneration. Symptoms such as flashing lights may indicate traction on the retina and impending retinal detachment. Difficulties with work, reading, watching television, and managing in the house should be identified. It is particularly important to assess the effect of the visual disability on the patient's lifestyle, especially as conditions such as cataracts can, with modern techniques, be operated on at an early stage.

The patient should also be asked exactly what is worrying them, as visual symptoms often cause great anxiety. Appropriate reassurance then can be given.

### Questions about particular symptoms

Some specific questions are important in certain circumstances. A history of ocular trauma or any high velocity injury—particularly a hammer and chisel injury—should suggest an intraocular foreign body. Other questions, for example about the type of discharge in a patient with a red eye, may enable you to make the diagnosis.

*Previous ocular history*
Easily forgotten, but essential. The patient's red eye may be associated with complications of contact lens wear—for example, allergy or a corneal abrasion or ulcer. A history of severe shortsightedness (myopia) considerably increases the risk of retinal detachment. A history of longsightedness (hypermetropia) and typically the use of reading glasses before the age of 40 increases the risk of angle closure glaucoma. Patients often forget to mention eye drops and eye operations if they are asked just about "drugs and operations." A purulent conjunctivitis requires much more urgent attention if the patient has previously had glaucoma drainage surgery, because of the risk of infection entering the eye.

*Medical history*
Many systemic disorders affect the eye, and the medical history may give clues to the cause of the problem; for instance, diabetes mellitus in a patient with a vitreous haemorrhage or sarcoidosis in a patient with uveitis.

*Family history*
A good example of the importance of the family history is in primary open angle glaucoma. This may be asymptomatic until severe visual damage has occurred. The risk of the disease may be as high as 1 in 10 in first degree relatives, and the disease may be arrested if treated at an early stage. For any disease that

---

**Visual symptoms: details to establish**
- Monocular or binocular
- Type of disturbance
- Rate of onset
- Presence and type of field loss
- Associated symptoms—for example, flashing lights or floaters
- Effect on lifestyle
- Specific worries

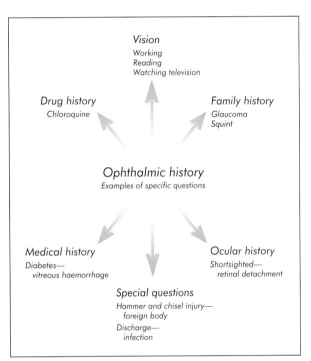

Answers to specific questions in the ophthalmic history will give clues to the diagnosis and help to exclude other problems

A history of a lazy eye (amblyopia) in a patient with a problem with their effective "only" eye is extremely important, as disturbance of vision in the good eye would result in definite functional impairment

A family history of glaucoma is a risk factor for the development of glaucoma

has a genetic component (for example, glaucoma), the age of onset and the severity of disease in affected family members can be very useful information.

*Drug history*

Many drugs affect the eye, and they should always be considered as a cause of ocular problems; for example, chloroquine may affect the retina. Steroid drugs in many different forms (drops, ointments, tablets, and inhalers) may all lead to steroid induced glaucoma.

---

**Assessment of vision**
- Snellen chart at 6 m
- Snellen chart closer
- Counting fingers
- Hand movements
- Perception of light
- No perception of light

---

# Examination of the visual system

## Vision

An assessment of visual acuity measures the function of the eye and gives some idea of the patient's disability. It may also have considerable medicolegal implications; for example, in the case of ocular damage at work or after an assault.

In the United Kingdom, visual acuity is checked with a standard Snellen chart at 6 m. If the room is not large enough, a mirror can be used with a reversed Snellen chart at 3 m. The numbers next to the letters indicate the distance at which a person with no refractive error can read that line (hence the 6/60 line should normally be read at 60 m). If the top line cannot be discerned, the test can be done closer to the chart. If the chart cannot be read at 1 m, patients may be asked to count fingers, and, if they cannot do that, to detect hand movements. Finally, it may be that they can perceive only light. From the patient's point of view, the functional difference between these categories may be the difference between managing at home on their own (count fingers) and total dependence on others (perception of light).

In other areas of the world (for example, the United States), visual acuity charts use a different nomenclature. Visual acuity of 20/20 is equivalent to 6/6 and 20/200 is equivalent to 6/60. A logarithmic chart (LogMAR) is also used, especially for large scale clinical trials and orthoptic childhood screening. The LogMAR system offers increased sensitivity in acuity testing, but the tests take longer to perform.

Vision should be tested with the aid of the patient's usual glasses or contact lenses. To achieve optimal visual acuity, the patient should be asked to look through a pinhole. This reduces the effect of any refractive error and particularly is useful if the patient cannot use contact lenses because of a red eye or has not brought their glasses. If patients cannot read English, they can be asked to match letters; this is also useful for young children.

Reading vision can be tested with a standard reading type book or, if this is not available, various sizes of newspaper print. There may be quite a difference in the near and distance vision. A good example is presbyopia, which usually develops in the late forties because of the failure of accommodation with age. Distance vision may be 6/6 without glasses, but the patient may be able to read only larger newspaper print.

Colour vision can be tested by using Ishihara colour plates, which may give useful information in cases of inherited and acquired abnormalities of colour vision. The ability to detect relative degrees of image contrast (contrast sensitivity) is also important and can be assessed with a Pelli-Robson chart. Some eye problems (such as cataract, for example) may cause a significant reduction in contrast sensitivity, despite good Snellen visual acuity.

## Field of vision

Tests of the visual field may give clues to the site of any lesion and the diagnosis. It is important to test the visual field in any

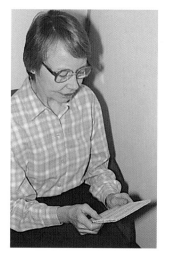
Testing reading vision

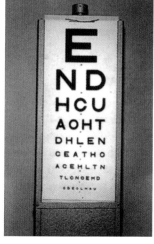
Visual acuity chart

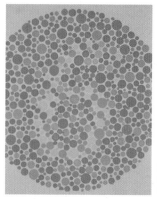
Ishihara colour plate. If a person is colour blind they cannot see the number

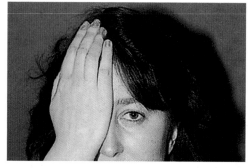
Testing the visual field. Ask the patient to cover the eye not being tested. Ensure that the eye is completely covered by the palm

patient with unexplained visual loss. Patients with lesions that affect the retrochiasmal visual pathway may find it difficult to verbalise exactly why their vision is "not right."

*Location of the lesion*—Unilateral field loss in the lower nasal field suggests an upper temporal retinal lesion. Central field loss usually indicates macular or optic nerve problems. A homonymous hemianopia or quadrantanopia indicates problems in the brain rather than the eye, although the patient may present with visual disturbance.

*Diagnosis*—A bitemporal field defect is most commonly caused by a pituitary tumour. A field defect that arches over central vision to the blind spot (arcuate scotoma) is almost pathognomonic of glaucoma.

*To test the visual field*—The patient should be seated directly opposite the examiner and then should be asked to cover the eye that is not being tested and to look at the examiner's face. It is essential to make sure that the other eye is covered properly to eliminate erroneous results. In case of a gross defect, the patient will not be able to see part of the examiner's face and may be able to indicate this precisely: "I can't see the centre of your face."

If no gross defect is present, the fields can be tested more formally. Testing the visual field with peripheral finger movements will show severe defects, but a more sensitive test is the detection of red colour, because the ability to detect red tends to be affected earlier. A red pin is moved in from the periphery and the patient is asked when they can see something red.

## The pupils

Careful inspection of the pupils can show signs that are helpful in diagnosis. A bright torch is essential. A pupil stuck down to the lens is a result of inflammation within the eye, which always is serious. A peaked pupil after ocular injury suggests perforation with the iris trapped in the wound. A vertically oval unreactive pupil may be seen in acute closed angle glaucoma.

The pupil's reaction to a good light source is a simple way of checking the integrity of the visual pathways. When testing the direct and consensual pupil reactions to light, the illumination in the room should be reduced and the patient should focus on a distant point. By the time pupils do not react to direct light, the damage is very severe. A much more sensitive test is the relative difference in pupillary reactions. Move the torchlight to and fro between the eyes, not allowing time for the pupils to dilate fully. If one of the pupils continues to dilate when the light shines on it, there is a defect in the visual pathway on that side (relative afferent pupillary defect). Cataracts and macular degeneration do not usually cause an afferent pupillary defect unless the lesions are particularly advanced. Neurological disease must be suspected.

Other important and potentially life threatening conditions in which the pupils are affected include Horner's syndrome, where the pupil is small but reactive with an associated ptosis. This condition may be caused by an apical lung carcinoma. The well known Argyll Robertson pupils caused by syphilis (bilateral small irregular pupils with light-near dissociation) are rare. In a third nerve palsy there is ptosis and the eye is divergent. The pupil size and reactions in such a case give important clues to the aetiology. If the pupil is unaffected ("spared"), the cause is likely to be medical—for example, diabetes or hypertension. If the pupil is dilated and fixed, the cause is probably surgical—for example, a treatable intracranial aneurysm.

Any differences in the colour of the two irides (heterochromia iridis) should be noted as this may indicate congenital Horner's syndrome, certain ocular inflammatory conditions (Fuch's heterochromic cyclitis), or an intraocular foreign body.

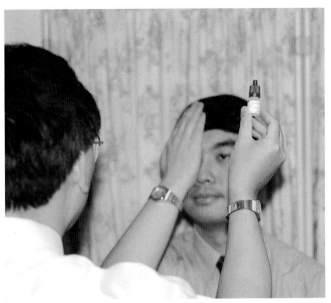

Using a readily available red target (for example, a tropicamide bottle top) to test the visual field

An extremely sensitive test of the fields is the comparison of the red in different quadrants. A good example is a patient who may have clinical signs of pituitary disease such as acromegaly; an early temporal defect can be detected if the patient is asked to *compare* the "quality" of the red colour in the upper temporal and nasal fields

Abnormal pupil reactions in the presence of ocular symptoms always should be treated seriously

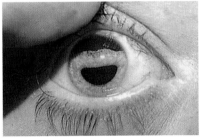

Torn peripheral iris (iridodialysis)

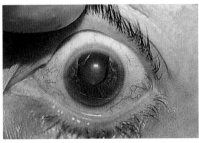

Distorted pupil after broad iridectomy

**Eye position and movements**

The appearance of the eyes shows the presence of any large degree of misalignment. This can, however, be misleading if the medial folds of the eyelids are wide. The position of the corneal reflections helps to confirm whether there is a true "squint." Squints and cover tests are dealt with in Chapter 11.

Patients should be asked if they have any double vision. If so, they should be asked to say whether diplopia occurs in any particular direction of gaze. It is important to exclude palsies of the third (eye turned out) or sixth (failure of abduction) cranial nerves, as these may be secondary to life threatening conditions. Complex abnormalities of eye movements should lead you to suspect myasthenia gravis or dysthyroid eye disease. The presence of nystagmus should be noted, as it may indicate significant neurological disease.

A protruding globe (proptosis) or a sunken globe (enophthalmos) should be recorded. Proptosis is always an important finding: its rate of onset and progression may give clues to the underlying pathology, and the direction of globe displacement indicates the site of the pathology.

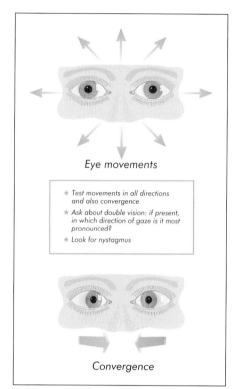

Eye movements

* Test movements in all directions and also convergence
* Ask about double vision: if present, in which direction of gaze is it most pronounced?
* Look for nystagmus

Convergence

Test eye movements in all directions and when converging

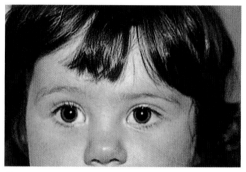

Normal position of corneal light reflexes

**Eyelids, conjunctiva, sclera, and cornea**

Examination of the eyelids, conjunctiva, sclera, and cornea should be performed in good light and with magnification. You will need:

* a bright torch (with a blue filter for use with fluorescein) or an ophthalmoscope with a blue filter
* a magnifying aid.

The lower lid should be gently pulled down to show the conjunctival lining and any secretions in the lower fornix.

The anterior chamber should be examined, looking specifically at the depth (a shallow anterior chamber is seen in angle-closure glaucoma and perforating eye injuries) and for the presence of pus (hypopyon) or blood (hyphaema). All these signs indicate serious disease that needs immediate ophthalmic referral.

If there are symptoms of "grittiness," a red eye or any history of foreign body, the upper eyelid should be everted.

**The cornea should be stained with fluorescein eye drops. If this is not done, many lesions, including large corneal ulcers, may be missed**

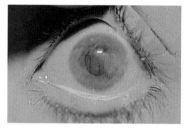

Corneal abrasion stained with fluorescein and illuminated with blue light

**Eyelids—Compare both sides and note position, lid lesions, and conditions of margins**

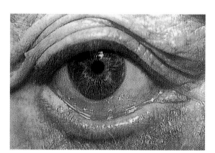

Ectropion

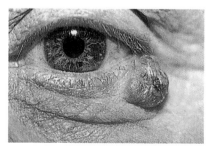

Basal cell carcinoma

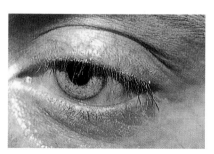

Blepharitis

This should not be done, however, if there is any question of ocular perforation, as the ocular contents may prolapse.

*Conjunctiva and sclera*—Look for local or generalised inflammation and pull down the lower lid and evert upper lid.

*Cornea*—Look at clarity and stain with fluorescein.

*Anterior chamber*—Check for blood and pus; also check chamber depth.

The drainage angle of the eye can be checked with a special lens (gonioscope).

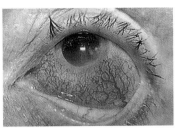

Scleritis: localised redness

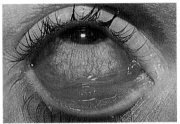

Conjunctivitis: generalised redness

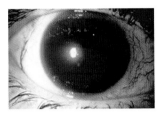

Blood in anterior chamber (hyphaema)

### Intraocular pressure

Assessment of intraocular pressure by palpation is useful only when the intraocular pressure is considerably raised, as in acute closed angle glaucoma. The eye should be gently palpated between two fingers and compared with the other eye or with the examiner's eye. The eye with acute glaucoma feels hard. Consider acute angle closure in any person over the age of 50 with a red eye.

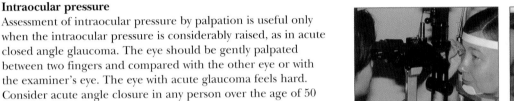

Special contact lens being used to view the drainage angle of the eye (gonioscope)

### Ophthalmoscopy

Good ophthalmoscopy is essential to avoid missing many serious ocular and general diseases. A direct ophthalmoscope can be used to allow intraocular structures to be seen. Specific contact and non-contact lenses are used during the examination, and the ophthalmologist should use a slit-lamp microscope or head-mounted ophthalmoscope.

To get a good view, the pupil should be dilated. There is an associated risk of precipitating acute angle closure glaucoma, but this is very small. The best dilating drop is tropicamide 1%, which is short acting and has little effect on accommodation. However, the effects may still last several hours, so the patient should be warned about this and told not to drive until any blurring of vision has subsided.

The direct ophthalmoscope should be set on the "0" lens. The patient should be asked to fix their gaze on an object in the distance, as this reduces pupillary constriction and accommodation, and helps keep the eye still. To enable a patient to fix on a distant object with the other eye, the examiner should use his right eye to examine the patient's right eye, and vice versa. The light should be shone at the eye until the red reflex is elicited. This red reflex is the reflection from the fundus and is best assessed from a distance of about 50 cm. If the red reflex is either absent or diminished, this indicates an opacity between the cornea and retina. The most common opacity is a cataract.

The optic disc should then be located and brought into focus with the lenses in the ophthalmoscope. If a patient has a high refractive error, they can be asked to leave their glasses on, although this can cause more reflections. The physical signs at the disc may be the only chance of detecting serious disease in the patient. The retina should be scanned for abnormalities such as haemorrhages, exudates, or new vessels. The green filter on the ophthalmoscope helps to enhance blood vessels and microaneurysms. Finally the macula should be examined

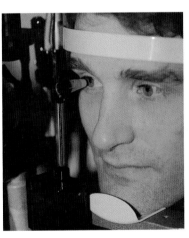

Measuring intraocular pressure by applanation tonometry

Patients should always be warned to seek help immediately if they have symptoms of pain or haloes around lights, after having their pupils dilated

for the pigmentary changes of age-related macular degeneration and the exudates of diabetic maculopathy.

It is viewed using a slit-lamp microscope and lens or head mounted indirect ophthalmoscope. However, these techniques are specialised.

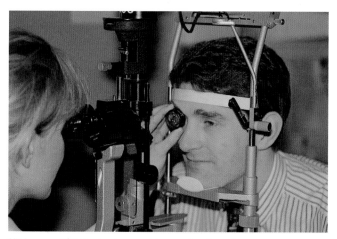

Slit-lamp and 78 dioptre lens used to examine the retina

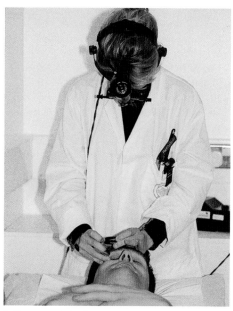

Indirect ophthalmoscopy

# Optic disc, retina, and macula

## Physical signs of disease at the disc

- A blurred disc edge may be the only sign of a cerebral tumour
- Cupping of the optic disc may be the only sign of undetected primary open angle glaucoma
- New vessels at the disc may herald blinding proliferative retinopathy in a patient without symptoms
- A pale disc may be the only stigma of past attacks of optic neuritis or of a compressive cerebral tumour

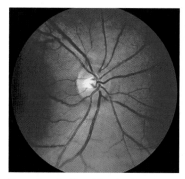

Normal optic disc with a healthy pink rim

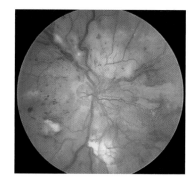

New vessels on optic disc in diabetes

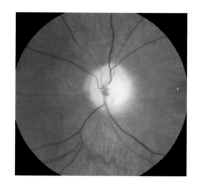

Optic atrophy—pale disc

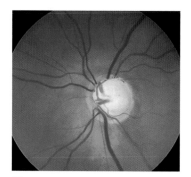

Glaucomatous cupping—displacement of vessels and pale disc

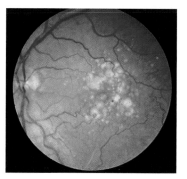

Age-related macular degeneration— deposits in macular area

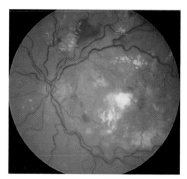

Diabetic maculopathy—oedema, exudates, and haemorrhages

# 2  Red eye

The "red eye" is one of the most common ophthalmic problems presenting to the general practitioner. An accurate history is important and should pay particular attention to vision, degree, and type of discomfort and the presence of a discharge. The history, and a good examination, will usually permit the diagnosis to be made without specialist ophthalmic equipment.

## Symptoms and signs

The most important symptoms are pain and visual loss; these suggest serious conditions such as corneal ulceration, iritis, and acute glaucoma. A purulent discharge suggests bacterial conjunctivitis; a clear discharge suggests a viral or allergic cause. A gritty sensation is common in conjunctivitis, but a foreign body must be excluded, particularly if only one eye is affected. Itching is a common symptom in allergic eye disease, blepharitis, and topical drop hypersensitivity.

**Corneal abrasions will be missed if fluorescein is not used**

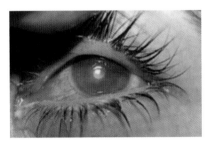

Corneal abscess (*Pseudomonas*) in contact lens wearer

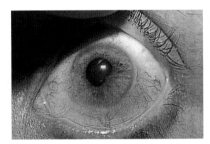

Anterior uveitis with ciliary flush around cornea and irregular stuck down pupil

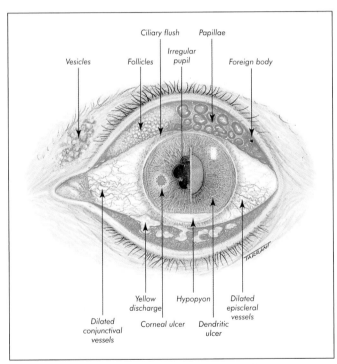

Important physical signs to look for in a patient with a red eye

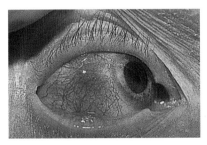

Scleritis—deeply injected and usually painful

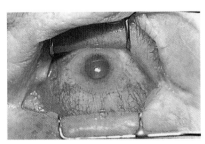

Acute angle closure glaucoma with red eye, semidilated pupil, and hazy cornea

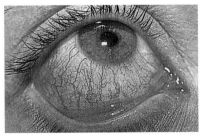

Bacterial conjunctivitis without discharge

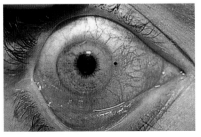

Foreign body

# Conjunctivitis

Conjunctivitis is one of the most common causes of an uncomfortable red eye. Conjunctivitis itself has many causes, including bacteria, viruses, *Chlamydia*, and allergies.

## Bacterial conjunctivitis

*History*—The patient usually has discomfort and a purulent discharge in one eye that characteristically spreads to the other eye. The eye may be difficult to open in the morning because the discharge sticks the lashes together. There may be a history of contact with a person with similar symptoms.

*Examination*—The vision should be normal after the discharge has been blinked clear of the cornea. The discharge usually is mucopurulent and there is uniform engorgement of all the conjunctival blood vessels. When fluorescein drops are instilled in the eye there is no staining of the cornea.

*Management*—Topical antibiotic eye drops (for example, chloramphenicol) should be instilled every two hours for the first 24 hours to hasten recovery, decreasing to four times a day for one week. Chloramphenicol ointment applied at night may also increase comfort and reduce the stickiness of the eyelids in the morning. Patients should be advised about general hygiene measures; for example, not sharing face towels.

## Viral conjunctivitis

Viral conjunctivitis commonly is associated with upper respiratory tract infections and is usually caused by an adenovirus. This is the type of conjunctivitis that occurs in epidemics of "pink eye."

*History*—The patient normally complains of both eyes being gritty and uncomfortable, although symptoms may begin in one eye. There may be associated symptoms of a cold and a cough. The discharge is usually watery.

Viral conjunctivitis usually lasts longer than bacterial conjunctivitis and may go on for many weeks; patients need to be informed of this. Photophobia and discomfort may be severe if the patient goes on to develop discrete corneal opacities.

*Examination*—Both eyes are red with diffuse conjunctival injection (engorged conjunctival vessels) and there may be a clear discharge. Small white lymphoid aggregations may be present on the conjunctiva (follicles). Small focal areas of corneal inflammation with erosions and associated opacities may give rise to pronounced symptoms, but these are difficult to see without high magnification. There may be associated head and neck lymphadenopathy with marked pre-auricular lymphadenopathy.

*Management*—Viral conjunctivitis is generally a self limiting condition, but antibiotic eye drops (for example, chloramphenicol) provide symptomatic relief and help prevent secondary bacterial infection. Viral conjunctivitis is extremely contagious, and strict hygiene measures are important for both the patient and the doctor; for example, washing of hands and sterilising of instruments. The period of infection is often longer than with bacterial pathogens and patients should be warned that symptoms may be present for several weeks. In some patients the infection may have a chronic, protracted course and steroid eye drops may be indicated if the corneal lesions and symptoms are persistent.

Steroids must only be prescribed with ophthalmological supervision, because of the real danger of causing cataract or irreversible glaucomatous damage. Furthermore, if long term steroids are required, patients should remain under continuous ophthalmological supervision.

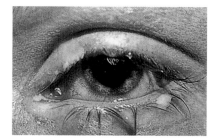

Purulent bacterial conjunctivitis

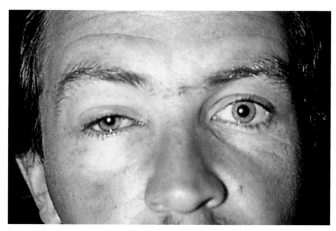

Adenovirus conjunctivitis of the right eye and enlarged preauricular nodes

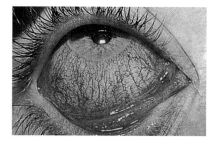

Viral conjunctivitis

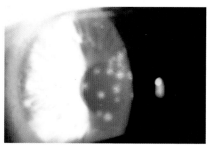

Chronic adenovirus infection

**Topical steroids should not be prescribed or continued without continuous ophthalmological supervision—potentially blinding complications may occur**

## Chlamydial conjunctivitis

*History*—Patients usually are young with a history of a chronic bilateral conjunctivitis with a mucopurulent discharge. There may be associated symptoms of venereal disease. Patients generally do not volunteer genitourinary symptoms when presenting with conjunctivitis; these need to be elicited through questioning.

*Examination*—There is bilateral diffuse conjunctival injection with a mucopurulent discharge. There are many lymphoid aggregates in the conjunctiva (follicles). The cornea usually is involved (keratitis) and an infiltrate of the upper cornea (pannus) may be seen.

*Management*—The diagnosis is often difficult and special bacteriological tests may be necessary to confirm the clinical suspicions. Treatment with oral tetracycline or a derivative for at least one month can eradicate the problem, but poor compliance can lead to a recurrence of symptoms. Systemic tetracycline can affect developing teeth and bones and should not be used in children or pregnant women.

Associated venereal disease should also be treated, and it is important to check the partner for symptoms or signs of venereal disease (affected females may be asymptomatic). It often is helpful to discuss cases with a genitourinary specialist before commencing treatment, so that all relevant microbiological tests can be performed at an early stage.

In developing countries, infection by *Chlamydia trachomatis* results in severe scarring of the conjunctiva and the underlying tarsal plate. These cicatricial changes cause the upper eyelids to turn in (entropion) and permanently scar the already damaged cornea. Worldwide, trachoma is still one of the major causes of blindness.

## Conjunctivitis in infants

Conjunctivitis in young children is extremely important because the eye defences are immature and a severe conjunctivitis with membrane formation and bleeding may occur. Serious corneal disease and blindness may result. **Conjunctivitis in an infant less than one month old (ophthalmia neonatorum) is a notifiable disease**. Such babies must be seen in an eye department so that special cultures can be taken and appropriate treatment given. Venereal disease in the parents must be excluded.

## Allergic conjunctivitis

*History*—The main feature of allergic conjunctivitis is itching. Both eyes usually are affected and there may be a clear discharge. There may be a family history of atopy or recent contact with chemicals or eye drops. Similar symptoms may have occurred in the same season in previous years. It is important to differentiate between an acute allergic reaction and a more long term chronic allergic eye disease.

*Examination*—The conjunctivae are diffusely injected and may be oedematous (chemosis). The discharge is clear and stringy. Because of the fibrous septa that tether the eyelid (tarsal) conjunctivae, oedema results in round swellings (papillae). When these are large they are referred to as cobblestones.

*Management*—Topical antihistamine and vasoconstrictor eye drops provide short term relief. Eye drops that prevent degranulation of mast cells also are useful, but they may need to be used for several weeks or months to achieve maximal effect. Oral antihistamines may also be used, particularly the newer compounds that cause less sedation. Topical steroids are effective but should not be used without regular ophthalmological supervision because of the risk of steroid induced cataracts and glaucoma, which may irreversibly

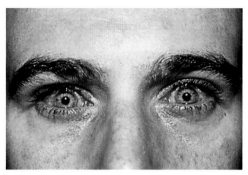
Chlamydial conjunctivitis—exclude associated venereal disease

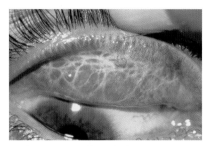
Trachoma—scarred tarsal plate

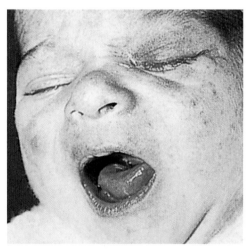
Infantile conjunctivitis—notifiable disease

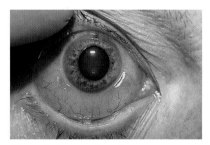
Chemosis due to pollen allergy

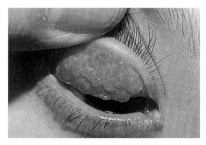
Large papillae in allergic conjunctivitis

damage vision. Cases of allergic eye disease in association with severe eczema will often need careful combined ophthalmological and dermatological management.

## Episcleritis and scleritis

Episcleritis and scleritis usually present as a localised area of inflammation. The episclera lies just beneath the conjunctiva and adjacent to the tough white scleral coat of the eye. Both the sclera and episclera may become inflamed, particularly in rheumatoid arthritis and other autoimmune conditions, but no cause is found for most cases of episcleritis.

*History*—The patient complains of a red and sore eye that may also be tender. There may be reflex lacrimation but usually there is no discharge. Scleritis is much more painful than episcleritis. The pain of scleritis often is sufficiently severe to wake the patient at night.

*Examination*—There is a localised area of inflammation that is tender to the touch. The episcleral and scleral vessels are larger than the conjunctival vessels. The signs of inflammation are usually more florid in scleritis.

*Management*—Any underlying cause should be identified. Episcleritis is essentially self limiting, but steroid eye drops hasten recovery and provide symptomatic relief. Scleritis is much more serious, and all patients need ophthalmological review. Serious systemic disorders need to be excluded, and systemic immunosuppressive treatment may be required.

## Corneal ulceration

Corneal ulcers may be caused by bacterial, viral, or fungal infections; these may occur as primary events or may be secondary to an event that has compromised the eye—for example, abrasion, wearing contact lenses, or use of topical steroids.

*History*—Pain usually is a prominent feature as the cornea is an exquisitely sensitive structure, although this is not so when corneal sensation is impaired; for example, after herpes zoster ophthalmicus. Indeed, this lack of sensory innervation may be the cause of the ulceration. There may be clues such as similar past attacks, facial cold sores, a recent abrasion, or the wearing of contact lenses.

*Examination*—Visual acuity depends on the location and size of the ulcer, and normal visual acuity does not exclude an ulcer. There may be a watery discharge due to reflex lacrimation or a mucopurulent discharge in bacterial ulcers. Conjunctival injection may be generalised or localised if the ulcer is peripheral, giving a clue to its presence. Fluorescein must be used or an ulcer easily may be missed. Certain types of corneal ulceration are characteristic; for example, dendritic lesions of the corneal epithelium usually are caused by infection with the herpes simplex virus. If there is inflammation in the anterior chamber there may be a collection of pus present (hypopyon). The upper eyelid must be everted or a subtarsal foreign body causing corneal ulceration may be missed. Patients with subtarsal foreign bodies sometimes do not recollect anything entering the eye.

*Management*—Patients with corneal ulceration should be referred urgently to an eye department or the eye may be lost. Management depends on the cause of the ulceration. The diagnosis usually will be made on the clinical appearance. The appropriate swabs and cultures should be arranged to try to identify the causative organism.

Intensive treatment then is started with drops and ointment of broad spectrum antibiotics until the organisms and their

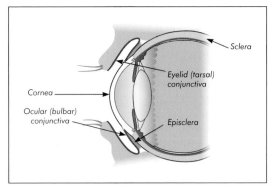

Conjunctiva, sclera, and episclera

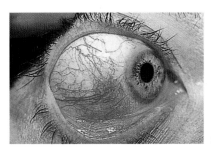

Episcleritis

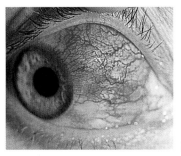

Scleritis

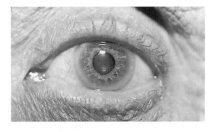

Eye with herpes simplex ulcer (not visible without fluorescein)

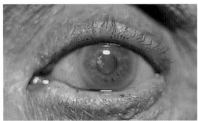

Same eye stained with fluorescein and viewed with blue light (ulcer visible)

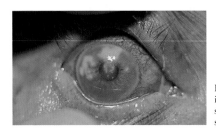

Herpes simplex ulcers inadvertently treated with steroids. Ulceration has spread and deepened

sensitivities to various antibiotics are known. Injections of antibiotics into the subconjunctival space may be given to increase local concentrations of the drugs.

Topical antiviral therapy should be used for herpetic infections of the cornea. Cycloplegic drops are used to relieve pain resulting from spasm of the ciliary muscle, and as they are also mydriatics they prevent adhesion of the iris to the lens (posterior synechiae). Topical steroids may be used to reduce local inflammatory damage not caused by direct infection, but the indications for their use are specific and they should not be used without ophthalmological supervision.

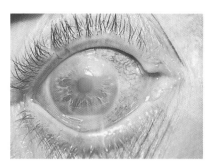

Corneal abscess with pus in anterior chamber (hypopyon)

# Iritis, iridocyclitis, anterior uveitis, and panuveitis

The iris, ciliary body, and choroid are similar embryologically and are known as the uveal tract. Inflammation of the iris (iritis) does not occur without inflammation of the ciliary body (cyclitis) and together these are referred to as iridocyclitis or anterior uveitis. Thus the terms are synonymous. It is important to consider diabetes mellitus in any patient with recent onset anterior uveitis.

Several groups of patients are at risk of developing anterior uveitis, including those who have had past attacks of iritis and those with a seronegative arthropathy, particularly if they are positive for the HLA B27 histocompatibility antigen; for example, a young man with ankylosing spondylitis. Children with seronegative arthritis are also at high risk, particularly if only a few joints (pauciarticular) are affected by the arthritis.

Uveitis in children with juvenile chronic arthritis may be relatively asymptomatic and they may suffer serious ocular damage if they are not screened. Sarcoidosis also causes chronic anterior uveitis, as do several other conditions including herpes zoster ophthalmicus, syphilis, and tuberculosis.

In panuveitis both the anterior and posterior segments of the eyes are inflamed and patients may have evidence of an associated systemic disease (for example, sarcoidosis, Behçet's syndrome, systemic lupus erythematosus, polyarteritis nodosa, Wegener's granulomatosis, or toxoplasmosis).

*History*—The patient who has had past attacks can often feel an attack coming on even before physical signs are present. There is often pain in the later stages, with photophobia due to inflammation and ciliary spasm. The pain may be worse when the patient is reading and contracting the ciliary muscle.

*Examination*—The vision initially may be normal but later it may be impaired. Accommodation, and hence reading vision, may be affected. There may be inflammatory cells in the anterior chamber, cataracts may form, and adhesions may develop between the iris and lens. The affected eye is red with the injection particularly being pronounced over the area that covers the inflamed ciliary body (ciliary flush). The pupil is small because of spasm of the sphincter, or irregular because of adhesions of the iris to the lens (posterior synechiae). An abnormal pupil in a red eye usually indicates serious ocular disease. Inflammatory cells may be deposited on the back of the cornea (keratitic precipitates) or may settle to form a collection of cells in the anterior chamber of the eye (hypopyon).

*Management*—If there is an underlying cause it must be treated, but in many cases no cause is found. It is important to ensure there is no disease in the rest of the eye that is giving rise to signs of an anterior uveitis, such as more posterior inflammation, a retinal detachment, or an intraocular tumour. Treatment is with topical steroids to reduce the inflammation

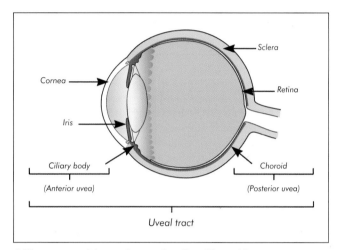

Different parts of the eye that may be affected by uveitis

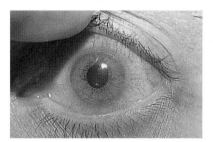

Anterior uveitis or iritis with ciliary flush but pupil not stuck down

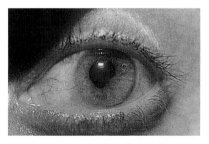

Anterior uveitis with ciliary flush and irregular pupil

and prevent adhesions within the eye. The ciliary body is paralysed to relieve pain, and the associated dilation of the pupil also prevents the development of adhesions between the iris and the lens that can cause "pupil block" glaucoma. The intraocular pressure may also rise because inflammatory cells block the trabecular meshwork, and antiglaucoma treatment may be needed if this occurs. Continued inflammation may lead to permanent damage of the trabecular meshwork and secondary glaucoma, cataracts, and oedema of the macula.

Patients with panuveitis will need systemic investigation and possibly systemic immunosuppression.

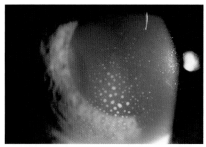

Keratic precipitates

## Acute angle closure glaucoma

Acute angle closure glaucoma always should be considered in a patient over the age of 50 with a painful red eye. The diagnosis must not be missed or the eye will be damaged permanently. The mechanism is dealt with in Chapter 9.

*History*—The attack usually comes on quite quickly, characteristically in the evening, when the pupil becomes semidilated. There is pain in one eye, which can be extremely severe and may be accompanied by vomiting. The patient complains of impaired vision and haloes around lights due to oedema of the cornea. The patient may have had similar attacks in the past which were relieved by going to sleep (the pupil constricts during sleep, so relieving the attack). The patient may have needed reading glasses earlier in life. A patient with acute angle closure glaucoma may be systemically unwell, with severe headache, nausea, and vomiting, and can be misdiagnosed as an acute abdominal or neurosurgical emergency. Acute angle closure glaucoma also may present in patients immediately postoperatively after general anaesthesia, and in patients receiving nebulised drugs (salbutamol and ipratropium bromide) for pulmonary disease.

*Examination*—The eye is inflamed and tender. The cornea is hazy and the pupil is semidilated and fixed. Vision is impaired according to the state of the cornea. On gentle palpation the eye feels harder than the other eye. The anterior chamber seems shallower than usual, with the iris being close to the cornea. If the patient is seen after the resolution of an attack the signs may have disappeared, hence the importance of the history.

*Management*—Urgent referral to hospital is required. Emergency treatment is needed if the sight of the eye is to be preserved. If it is not possible to get the patient to hospital straight away, intravenous acetazolamide 500 mg should be given, and pilocarpine 4% should be instilled in the eye to constrict the pupil.

First the pressure must be brought down medically and then a hole made in the iris with a laser (iridotomy) or surgically (iridectomy) to restore normal aqueous flow. The other eye should be treated prophylactically in a similar way. If treatment is delayed, adhesions may form between the iris and the cornea (peripheral anterior synechiae) or the trabecular meshwork may be irreversibly damaged necessitating a full surgical drainage procedure.

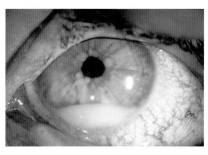

Hypopyon uveitis

### Features of acute angle closure glaucoma

- Pain
- Haloes around lights
- Impaired vision
- Fixed semidilated pupil
- Hazy cornea
- Age more than 50
- Eye feels hard
- Unilateral

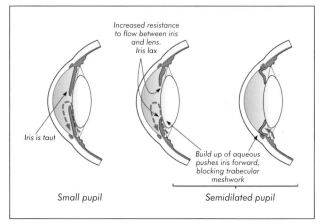

Acute angle closure glaucoma. Note the corneal oedema (irregular reflected image of light on cornea) and fixed semidilated pupil

Increased resistance to flow between iris and lens. Iris lax

Iris is taut

Build up of aqueous pushes iris forward, blocking trabecular meshwork

Small pupil

Semidilated pupil

Acute angle closure glaucoma

## Subconjunctival haemorrhage

*History*—The patient usually presents with a red eye which is comfortable and without any visual disturbance. It is usually the appearance of the eye that has made the patient seek attention. If there is a history of trauma, or a red eye after hammering or chiselling, then ocular injury and an intraocular foreign body must be excluded. Subconjunctival haemorrhages are often seen on the labour ward post partum.

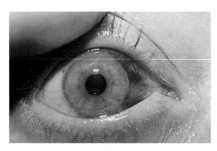

Subconjunctival haemorrhage

*Examination*—There is a localised area of subconjunctival blood that is usually relatively well demarcated. There is no discharge or conjunctival reaction. Look for skin bruising and evidence of a blood dyscrasia.

*Management*—It is worth checking the blood pressure to exclude hypertension. If there are no other abnormalities the patient should be reassured and told the redness may take several weeks to fade. If patients are anticoagulated with warfarin then the coagulation profile (international normalised ratio, INR) should be checked. If abnormal bruising of the skin is present then consider checking the full blood count and platelets.

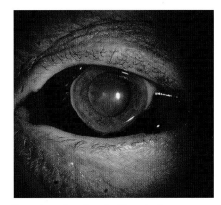
Extensive subconjunctival haemorrhage

# Inflamed pterygium and pingueculum

*History*—The patient complains of a focal red area or lump in the interpalpebral area. There may have been a pre-existing lesion in the area that the patient may have noticed before.

*Examination*—Pinguecula are degenerative areas on the conjunctiva found in the 4 and 8 o'clock positions adjacent to, but not invading, the cornea. These common lesions may be related to sun and wind exposure. Occasionally they become inflamed or ulcerated. A pterygium is a non-malignant fibrovascular growth that encroaches onto the cornea.

*Management*—If the pingueculum is ulcerated, antibiotics may be indicated. For a pterygium, surgical excision is indicated if it is a cosmetic problem, causes irritation, or is encroaching on the visual axis. Symptomatic relief from the associated tear-film irregularities are often helped by the use of topical artificial tear eye drops.

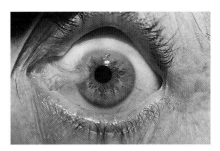
Pterygium

# Red eye that does not get better

Red eyes are so common that every doctor will be faced with a patient whose red eye does not improve with basic management. It is important to be aware of some of the more common differential diagnoses.

Many of the conditions described below will need a detailed ophthalmic assessment to make the diagnosis. Consider early ophthalmic referral when patients present with red eyes and atypical clinical features or fail to improve with basic management.

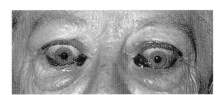
Bilaterial thyroid eye disease with exophthalmos and conjunctival oedema (chemosis)

### Orbital problems

It is easy to miss someone with early thyroid eye disease and patients can present with one or both eyes affected. Look for associated ocular (for example, lid retraction) and systemic features of thyroid disease. There are several rare but important orbital causes of chronic red eyes, including carotico-cavernous fistula, orbital inflammatory disease, and lymphoproliferative diseases.

### Eyelid problems

Malpositions of the eyelids such as entropion and ectropion often cause chronic conjunctival injection. Nasolacrimal obstruction presents with a watery eye but there can be chronic ocular injection if the cause is lacrimal canaliculitis or a lacrimal sac abscess. A periocular lid malignancy such as basal cell carcinoma or sebaceous (meibomian) gland carcinoma may rarely present as a unilateral chronic red eye.

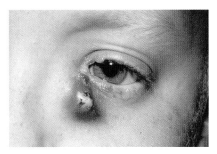
Acute dacrocystitis

### Conjunctival problems

If a patient has a history of an infective conjunctivitis that does not improve, then you should always exclude chlamydial conjunctivitis, particularly if there are also genitourinary

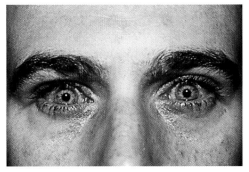
Chlamydial conjunctivitis

symptoms. Giant papillary conjunctivitis may occur in patients with ocular allergic disease or in contact lens wearers. If someone is on long term topical drug therapy (for example, for glaucoma) then drug hypersensitivity should be considered, especially if drug instillation causes marked itching or the eyelids have an eczematous appearance. Other causes of chronic red eyes include a subtarsal foreign body, dry eyes, and cicatricial ocular pemphigoid.

### Corneal problems

Corneal causes of a chronically red and irritated eye include loose corneal sutures (previous cataract or corneal graft surgery), herpetic keratitis, exposure keratitis (for example, in Bell's palsy), contact lens related keratitis, marginal keratitis (for example, in patients with blepharitis or rosacea), and corneal abscess. Fluorescein drops will reveal corneal staining in patients whose red eye syndrome is caused by a corneal problem.

### Viral infection

Adenoviral keratoconjunctivitis may lead to a red, painful eye for many weeks and patients should be warned of this. Patients with refractory adenoviral keratitis may occasionally need topical steroid therapy. This should only be undertaken with close ophthalmological supervision as it can be hard to wean patients off steroids.

### Scleral problems

Episcleritis and scleritis present with red eyes that do not respond to topical antibiotic therapy. Think of scleritis in any patient presenting with marked ocular pain and injection.

### Anterior chamber problems

Failure to consider uveitis in a patient with a red eye, photophobia, and pain can result in delays that make subsequent management more difficult. Angle closure glaucoma has a very characteristic clinical presentation that is easy to miss.

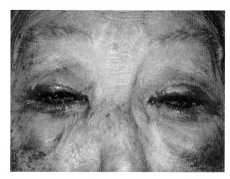

Drug hypersensitivity

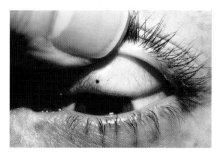

Subtarsal foreign body

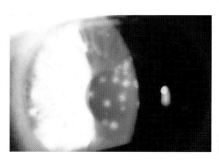

Chronic adenovirus infection

# 3  Refractive errors

Indistinct vision most commonly is caused by errors of refraction. Doctors do not often have to deal with this problem because patients usually are prescribed glasses by an optometrist. However, if a patient presents complaining of visual problems, it is extremely important to ask the question: "Is this patient's poor vision caused by a refractive error?"

The use of a simple "pinhole" made in a piece of card will help to determine whether or not there is a refractive error. In the absence of disease the vision will improve when the pinhole is used—unless the refractive error is extremely large.

## Eye with no refractive error

In an eye with no refractive error (emmetropia) light rays from infinity are brought to a focus on the retina by the cornea and lens when the eye is in a "relaxed" state. The cornea contributes about two thirds and the lens about one third to the eye's refractive power. Disease affecting the cornea (for example, keratoconus) may cause severe refractive problems.

The rays of light from closer objects, such as the printed page, are divergent and have to be brought to a focus on the retina by the process of accommodation. The circular ciliary muscle contracts, allowing the naturally elastic lens to assume a more globular shape that has a greater converging power.

In young people the lens is very elastic, but with age the lens gradually hardens and even when the ciliary muscle contracts the lens no longer becomes globular. Thus from the age of 40 onwards close work becomes gradually more difficult (presbyopia). Objects may have to be held further away to reduce the need for accommodation, which leads to the complaint "my arms don't seem to be long enough." Fine detail cannot be discerned.

Convex lenses in the form of reading glasses therefore are needed to converge the light rays from close objects on to the retina.

> **All emmetropic people need reading glasses for close work in later life**

People who wear glasses to see clearly in the distance may find it convenient to change to bifocal lenses in their glasses when they become presbyopic. In bifocal lenses the reading lens simply is incorporated into the lower part of the lens. Therefore, the person does not have to change his or her glasses to read. However, details at an intermediate distance such as the prices of items on supermarket shelves are not clear. A third lens segment can be incorporated between that for distance above and that for reading below, creating a trifocal lens. However, many people cannot cope with the "jump" in magnification inherent in the use of these lenses. This has led to the introduction of multifocal lenses in which the lens power increases progressively from top to bottom. People may also have problems adapting to this type of lens, as peripheral vision may be distorted.

Refractive errors do not get worse if a person reads in bad light or does not wear their glasses. The exceptions are young children, however, who may need a refractive error corrected to prevent amblyopia.

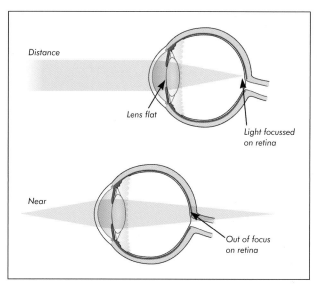

Eye with no refractive error. Light rays from distant objects are focused on to the retina without the need for accommodation. Light rays from a close object (for example, a book) are focused behind the retina. The eye has to accommodate to focus these rays

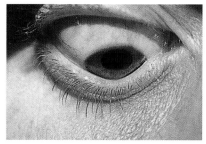

Conical cornea (keratoconus) indenting lower lid on down gaze

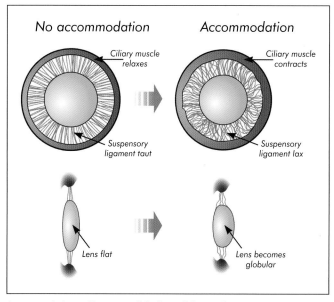

Accommodation: adjustment of the lens of the eye for viewing objects at various distances

# Myopic or shortsighted eye

In the myopic eye, light rays from infinity are brought to a focus in front of the retina because either the eye is too long or the converging power of the cornea and lens is too great. To achieve clear vision the rays of light must be diverged by a concave lens so that light rays are focused on the retina.

For near vision, light rays are focused on the retina with little or no accommodation depending on the degree of myopia and the distance at which the object is held. This is the reason why shortsighted people can often read without glasses even late in life, when those without refractive errors need reading glasses.

A certain type of cataract (nuclear sclerosis) increases the refractive power of the lens, making the eye more myopic. Patients with these cataracts may say their reading vision has improved. Patients with an extreme degree of shortsightedness are more susceptible to retinal detachment, macular degeneration, and primary open angle glaucoma.

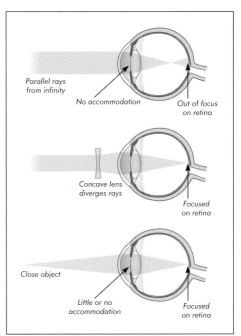

**Myopic or shortsighted eye.** Light rays from distant objects are focused in front of the retina, and the lens cannot compensate for this. A concave lens has to be placed in front of the eye to focus the rays on the retina. Light rays from close objects are focused on the retina with little or no accommodation. Thus, even with loss of accommodation, the myopic eye can read without glasses

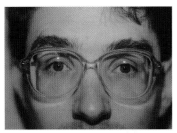

Myopic glasses: the face and eyes seem smaller behind the lenses

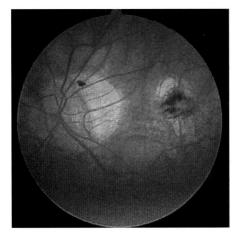

Macular degeneration with myopic crescent temporal to disc

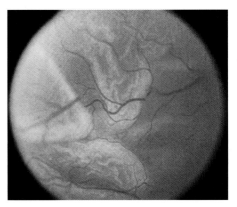

Retinal detachment

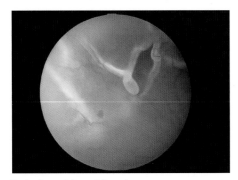

Retinal tear (about 0.5 mm)

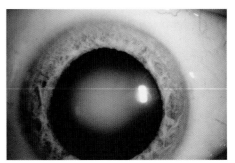

Nuclear sclerosis

# Hypermetropic or longsighted eye

In the hypermetropic eye, light rays from infinity are brought to a focus behind the retina, either because the eye is too short or because the converging power of the cornea and lens is too weak. Unlike the young shortsighted person, the young longsighted person can achieve a clear retinal image by accommodating. Extremely good distance vision can often be achieved by this "fine tuning"—for example, 6/4 on the Snellen chart—and this has given rise to the term "longsighted." For near vision the longsighted person has to accommodate even more. This may be possible during the first two to three decades of life, but the need for reading glasses arises earlier than in the normal person.

As the ability to accommodate (and thus compensate for the hypermetropia) fails with advancing years, the longsighted person may require glasses for both distant and near vision when none were needed before. This may result in the complaint of a deterioration in eyesight because the patient has gone from not needing glasses to needing them for both distance and near vision.

Longsighted people are more susceptible to closed angle glaucoma because their smaller eyes are more likely to have shallow anterior chambers and narrow angles.

# Astigmatic eye

Astigmatism occurs when the cornea does not have an even curvature. A good analogy is that of a soccer ball (no astigmatism) and a rugby ball (astigmatism). The curvature of a normal cornea may be likened to that of the back of a ladle and that of the astigmatic eye to the back of a spoon. This uneven curvature results in an uneven focus in different meridians, and the eye cannot compensate by accommodating.

Astigmatism can be corrected by a lens that has power in only one meridian (a cylinder). Alternatively, an evenly curved surface may be achieved by fitting a hard contact lens. Astigmatism can be caused by any disease that affects the shape of the cornea; for example, a meibomian cyst may press hard enough on the cornea to cause distortion.

> **Astigmatism can be measured by analysing the image of a series of concentric rings reflected from the cornea**

# Contact lenses

Contact lenses have become increasingly popular in recent years. There are several types, which can be grouped into three categories.

- *Hard lenses* are made of polymethylmethacrylate (plastic material) and are not permeable to gases or liquids. They cannot be worn continuously because the cornea becomes hypoxic and they are the most difficult lenses to get used to. Because of their rigidity, however, they correct astigmatism well and are durable. Infection and allergy are less likely with this type of lens. They are now less commonly prescribed, but there are still many people who have been using this type of lens for a long time with no problems.
- *Gas permeable lenses* have properties between those of hard and soft lenses. They allow the passage of oxygen through to the tear film and cornea, and they are better tolerated than hard lenses. Being semi-rigid they correct astigmatism better than soft lenses. They are, however, more prone to the accumulation of deposits and are also less durable than hard

> **Typically, the longsighted person needs reading glasses at about 30 years of age. If a high degree of hypermetropia is present, accommodation may not be adequate, and glasses may have to be worn for both distant and near vision from an earlier age**

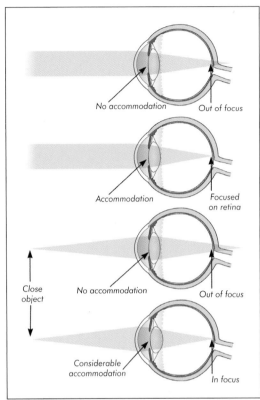

**Hypermetropic or longsighted eye.** Light rays from close objects are focused behind the retina. The considerable accommodation required is possible in a young person, but reading glasses are needed in later life

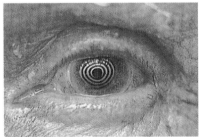

Reflections of concentric circles showing distortion by astigmatic cornea

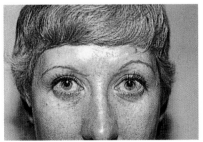

Gas permeable lenses to correct myopia

17

lenses. Gas permeable lenses usually are used as daily wear lenses.

- *Soft lenses* have a high water content and are permeable to both gases and liquids. They are tolerated much better than hard or gas permeable lenses and they can be worn for much longer periods. Both infection and allergy, however, are more common. The lenses are less durable, are more prone to the accumulation of deposits, and do not correct astigmatism as well as the harder lenses. Nevertheless, because they are so well tolerated, they are the most commonly prescribed lenses.

Certain types of gas permeable and soft lenses can be worn continuously for up to several months because of their high oxygen permeability, but the risk of sight threatening complications is higher than with daily wear lenses.

Disposable lenses are soft lenses that are designed to be thrown away after a short period of continuous use. They are popular because no cleaning is required during this period. However, it is important that the lenses are used as recommended, or the risk of complications, such as corneal infection, rise substantially.

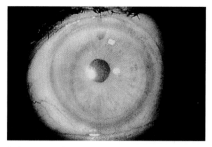
Soft contact lens fitted after cataract extraction

### Indications for prescribing contact lenses

Personal appearance and the inconvenience of spectacles are common reasons for prescribing contact lenses. They also may considerably reduce the optical aberrations that are associated with the wearing of glasses, particularly those with high power that are sometimes prescribed for patients who have had cataracts removed. The brain cannot resolve the large difference in the size of the retinal images that occurs when the refractive power of the two eyes differs considerably. For example, this occurs when a cataract has been removed from one eye and a spectacle lens has been prescribed but the other eye is normal. A contact lens brings the image size closer to "normal," permitting the brain to fuse the two images. If a person is very myopic, the use of contact lenses rather than spectacles may increase the image size on the retina and improve the visual acuity.

A contact lens can also neutralise irregularities in the cornea and correct the effects of an irregularly shaped cornea (for example, keratoconus or that which occurs after corneal graft surgery).

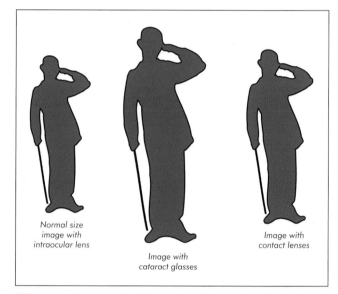

Normal size image with intraocular lens

Image with cataract glasses

Image with contact lenses

Different sized images with different types of optical correction after cataract surgery

### Relative contraindications to contact lens wear

Contraindications include a history of atopy, "dry eyes," previous glaucoma filtration surgery, and an inability to handle or cope with the management of lenses. These are, however, relative contraindications; a trial of lenses may be the only way to determine whether it is feasible for a particular patient to wear contact lenses.

---

**Contact lens wear—relative contradictions**
- Atopy
- Dry eyes
- Inability to insert, remove, and care for lenses

---

### Complications of wearing contact lenses

The most serious complication of contact lens wear is a corneal abscess. This is most common in elderly patients who have worn soft contact lenses for an extended period. Certain bacterial pathogens such as pneumococci or *Pseudomonas* species can cause severe corneal damage and even perforation. Other pathogens such as acanthamoebae can contaminate contact lenses or contact lens cases and can produce a chronic corneal infection with severe pain. Acanthamoebae live in tap water and it is important to instruct all contact lens wearers to avoid rinsing their lens cases with tap water. Corneal abrasions are also fairly common. Chronic lens overuse can lead to ingrowth of blood vessels into the normally avascular cornea.

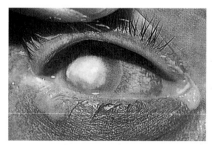
Corneal abscess associated with contact lens wear

Any contact lenses wearer with a red eye should have the contact lens removed and the eye stained with fluorescein to show up any corneal abrasion or abscess. **As fluorescein stains soft contact lenses, the eye should be washed out with saline before the lens is replaced**. If there is an abrasion or infection the appropriate treatment should be given, and the contact lens **should not be worn again** until the condition has resolved. The wearing time may have to be built up again, particularly if hard or gas permeable lenses are worn.

Good hygiene is essential for contact lens wearers, to minimise the risks of infection. Lenses should never be licked and replaced in the eye. Non-sterile solutions may contain contaminants such as amoebae, which can lead to intractable ocular infection.

# Refractive surgery

There has been much interest in operations to alter the refractive state of the eye, particularly operations to treat myopia. The technique called radial keratotomy entails making deep radial incisions in the peripheral cornea, which results in flattening of the central cornea and refocusing of light rays nearer the retina. It is only of use in short sight, and possible disadvantages include weakening of the cornea (particularly if the eye subsequently sustains trauma), infection, glare, and fluctuation of the refractive state of the eye. If contact lenses are still required after radial keratotomy has been performed, they are much more difficult to fit.

### Surface-photorefractive keratectomy (S-PRK)

A special (excimer) laser has been used to reprofile the surface of the cornea. This laser works by vaporising a very thin layer of the corneal stroma after the corneal epithelium has been debrided (photoablation), which reshapes the front surface of the cornea, changing its focusing power. This technique, known as surface-photorefractive keratectomy (S-PRK), is safer than radial keratotomy, as it does not involve deep cuts into the eye. Side effects include:

- *pain* for a few days after the laser treatment
- *haze-regression reactions* (a period when the vision becomes hazy, along with a tendency for the refraction to regress back towards myopia again)
- *overcorrection* with a hypermetropic shift (often poorly tolerated)
- *corneal opacification* caused by scarring of the treated zone, which may result in a reduction of best corrected visual acuity (usually transient) and glare.

Predictability of the final refractive result is poorer if the patient is very shortsighted. (This is particularly the case if the patient has more than 6 dioptres of myopia.)

### Laser assisted in situ keratomileusis (LASIK)

More recently, a technique called laser assisted in situ keratomileusis (LASIK) has been introduced. This entails cutting a superficial hinged flap in the cornea (about 160 to 200 μm thick) with an automated microkeratome, carrying out excimer laser reshaping of the underlying corneal stroma, and then replacing the flap. Advantages of the technique over surface laser treatment include more rapid stabilisation of vision, reduced corneal scarring (with a definite reduction in haze-regression reactions), and much better correction of higher degrees of myopia. Accuracy of LASIK is optimal up to −6.00 dioptre sphere (DS), good up to −8.00 DS, and starts to become increasingly less accurate over −10.00 DS.

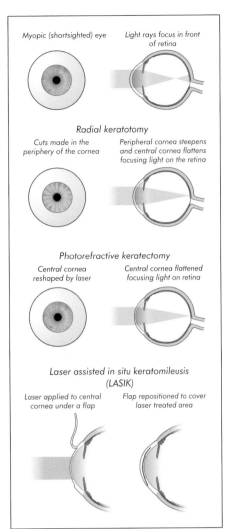

Different types of refractive surgery to correct myopia

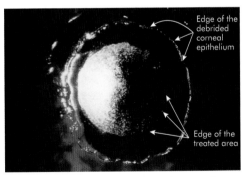

Surface-photorefractive keratectomy—the corneal epithelium has been removed and the laser has remodelled a precise area of the corneal stroma

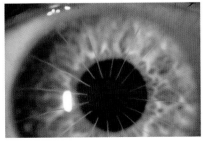

Radial keratotomy—the cornea is flattened by multiple radial incisions reducing the myopia

Disadvantages include complications associated with the technical difficulties of cutting and replacing the thin surface flap, which occur in 1–5% of patients.

A recent modification of LASIK is LASEK, in which an epithelial flap is raised prior to stromal ablation and then replaced. Other methods of altering the refractive status of the eye include corneal intrastromal rings, phakic intraocular lenses (intraocular lenses when the natural lens remains), and small incision clear lensectomy. Laser techniques can also be used to correct astigmatism and hypermetropia, although these are used much less commonly.

## Possible complications of surgery

Patients who are contemplating any type of refractive surgery should be fully informed of the risks by the operating surgeon and given time to evaluate the advantages and disadvantages before undergoing a procedure that may cause irreversible change. This is especially important as many patients will have pre-operative best corrected visual acuities of 6/6 or better (although they will need glasses or contact lenses to achieve this vision). It should be emphasised that the risk of complications is low, but complications are potentially devastating to vision. Complications that may occur include:

- *infection*—corneal infection is a rare problem associated with all refractive procedures and can substantially reduce vision.
- *corneal perforation*—this may very rarely occur in association with technical problems with the microkeratome in LASIK.
- *corneal flap problems*—there may occasionally be problems in cutting or replacing the corneal flap in LASIK. Flap irregularites, subflap foreign bodies, unstable flaps, and flap melts all have been reported. Epithelial ingrowth under the corneal flap is a rare complication.
- *corneal ectasia*—photoablative procedures all reduce the corneal thickness. If too much corneal stroma is removed then the cornea can progressively thin and become ectatic.
- *regression of refractive outcome*—in some patients the cornea undergoes a period of remodelling after refractive surgery, with a tendency to drift back towards the original refractive status.
- *refractive under- or overcorrection*—this occurs where the anticipated refractive correction does not occur. Overcorrection of myopia to produce hypermetropia often is tolerated poorly by the patient.
- *corneal stromal scarring*—postoperative corneal stromal scarring produces corneal haze, which produces optical aberrations (reduced best acuity, glare, reduced contrast, and problems with night vision).
- *optic neuropathy*—very rarely, patients have been reported to lose vision as a result of optic nerve damage after refractive procedures involving cutting a corneal flap. Optic nerve damage may be related to the transient but very high rise in intraocular pressure that occurs when the microkeratome is applied to the eye.
- *retinal detachment*—this serious complication may possibly be caused by tractional forces exerted on the eye when the microkeratome is used during refractive surgery.

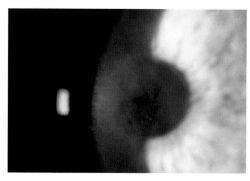

Grey scar in the corneal area treated by the laser

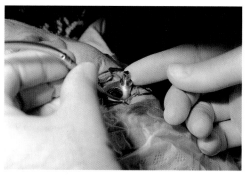

Microkeratome

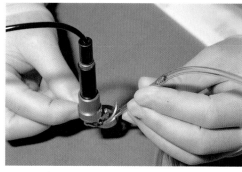

Microkeratome on eye

# 4   Eyelid, orbital, and lacrimal disorders

## Lumps in the lid

The most common lump found in the eyelid is a chalazion, but the accurate diagnosis of a lid lump is important because the lump may:

- *necessitate a disfiguring operation if not treated early*—basal cell carcinoma
- *be life threatening*—a deeply invading basal cell carcinoma
- *be the cause of visual disturbance*—a chalazion pressing on the cornea and causing astigmatism
- *indicate systemic disease*—xanthelasmas in a patient with hyperlipidaemia
- *cause amblyopia*—if it obstructs vision in a young child.

### Chalazion

A chalazion (meibomian cyst) is a granuloma of the lipid-secreting meibomian glands that lie in the lid. It is probably the result of a blocked duct, with local reaction to the accumulation of lipid.

The patient may initially complain of a lump in the lid that is hard and inflamed. This settles and the patient is left with a discrete lump in the lid that may cause astigmatism and consequent blurring of vision. Clinically there is a hard lump in the lid, which is clearly visible when the lid is everted.

Many chalazia settle on conservative treatment. This comprises warm compresses (with a towel soaked in warm water) and the application of chloramphenicol ointment. However if the chalazion is uncomfortable, excessively large, persistent, or disturbs vision, it can be incised and curetted under local anaesthesia from the inner conjunctival side of the eyelid.

Recurrent chalazia may indicate an underlying problem such as blepharitis, a skin disorder such as acne rosacea, or even, though very rarely, a malignant tumour of the meibomian glands.

### Stye

A stye and chalazion are often confused. A stye is an infection of a lash follicle, which causes a red, tender swelling at the lid margin. Unlike a chalazion, a stye may have a "head" of pus at the lid margin. It should be treated with warm compresses to help it to discharge, and chloramphenicol ointment should be used.

### Marginal cysts

Marginal cysts may develop from the lipid and sweat secreting glands around the margins of the eyelids. They are dome shaped with no inflammation. The cysts of the sweat glands are filled with clear fluid (cyst of Moll) and the cysts of the lipid secreting glands are filled with yellowish contents (cyst of Zeiss).

No treatment is indicated for marginal cysts that cause no problems. If they are a cosmetic blemish they can be removed under local anaesthesia.

### Papilloma

Papillomas are often pedunculated and multilobular. They are common and may be caused by viruses. They should be removed if they are large and the diagnosis is uncertain, or if they are disfiguring.

---

**Importance of lumps in the eyelid**
- May need disfiguring operations if left
- May be life threatening
- May be the cause of visual disturbance
- May cause blindness in children
- May indicate systemic disease

---

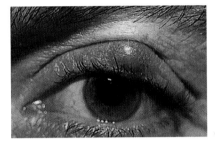

Chalazion

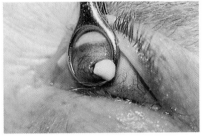

Incised chalazion

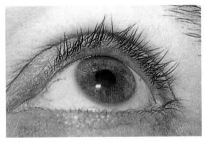

Stye

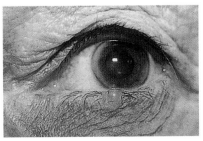

Cyst of sweat secreting gland (cyst of Moll)

21

### Xanthelasma

Xanthelasmas may be an incidental finding, or the patient may complain of yellow plaques on the nasal sides of the eyelids; these contain lipid. Associated hyperlipidaemia must be excluded and the lesions may be removed under local anaesthesia if they are a cosmetic problem.

### Basal cell carcinoma

Basal cell carcinoma (rodent ulcer) is the most common malignant tumour of the eyelid. It occurs mainly in the lower lid, which is particularly exposed to sunlight. The tumour does not metastasise but may be life threatening if allowed to infiltrate locally. Tumours in the medial canthal region may infiltrate the orbit extensively if they are not detected and dealt with. If the tumour is large when the patient is referred, an extensive and often disfiguring operation may be necessary.

The classical basal cell carcinoma has a pearly rounded edge with a necrotic centre, but it may be difficult to diagnose if it presents as a diffuse indurated lesion. It is particularly easy to miss the invasive form that occurs in a skin crease, which may be invading deeply with few cutaneous signs.

The patient should be referred urgently if there is any suspicion of a basal cell carcinoma. It usually is excised under local anaesthesia, unless complicated plastic reconstructive surgery is required. Radiotherapy may also be used as palliative therapy in periorbital disease. Patients with basal cell carcinomas around the eye will often have other facial skin tumours. Squamous cell carcinomas are rare in the periorbital region, but are much more locally invasive and may also metastasise.

# Inflammatory disease of the eyelid

### Blepharitis

Blepharitis is a common condition but is often not diagnosed. It is a chronic disease; the patient complains of persistently sore eyes. The symptoms may be intermittent and include a gritty sensation and sore eyelids. The patient may present with a chalazion or stye, which are much more common in patients with blepharitis, and these may be recurrent. Physical signs include inflamed lid margins, blocked meibomian gland orifices, and crusts round the lid margins. The conjunctiva may be inflamed, and punctate staining of the cornea may be visible on staining with fluorescein. Associated skin diseases include rosacea, eczema, and psoriasis. The aims of treatment are to:

- *keep the lids clean*—the crusts and coagulated lipid should be gently cleaned with a cotton wool bud dipped in warm water. This can be combined with baby shampoo to help remove lipid
- *treat infection*—antibiotic ointment should be smeared on the lid margin to help kill the staphylococci in the lid that may be aggravating the condition. This may be done for several months
- *replace tears*—the tear film in patients with blepharitis is abnormal, and artificial tears may provide considerable relief of symptoms
- *treat sebaceous gland dysfunction*—in severe cases, or those associated with sebaceous gland dysfunction, such as rosacea, oral tetracycline may be invaluable. Indications for referral are poor response to treatment and corneal disease.

### Acute inflammation of the eyelid

It is important to achieve a diagnosis in a patient with an acutely inflamed eyelid, as some conditions may be blinding—for example, orbital cellulitis (see page 25).

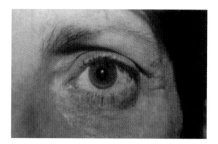

Xanthelasmas and corneal arcus in a young patient

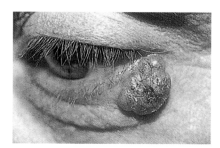

Basal cell carcinoma. Recently enlarging, with some bleeding

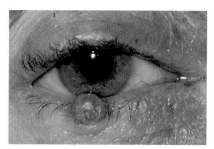

Basal cell carcinoma with classic pearly rolled edge

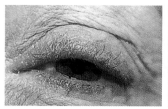

Blepharitis. Left: inflamed lid margin. Right: crust around lid margin

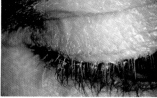

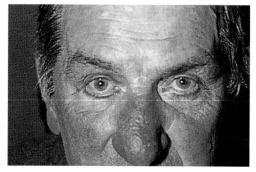

Rosacea with associated blepharitis

*Chalazion and stye*
Routine treatment should be given for these conditions. If infection is spreading, prescribe systemic antibiotics.

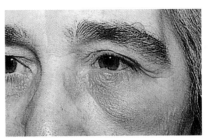

Chalazion with associated inflammation of the lower eyelid

*Spread of local infection*
Infection may have spread from a local lesion such as a "squeezed" comedo. Again, if there is spread of infection, systemic antibiotics are needed.

*Acute dacryocystitis*
The site of the inflammation is medial, over the lacrimal sac. There may be a history of previous watering of the eye as a result of a blocked lacrimal system that has since become infected. Treatment is with topical chloramphenicol and systemic antibiotics until the infection resolves. Recurrent attacks of dacryocystitis or symptomatic watering of the eye are indications for operation.

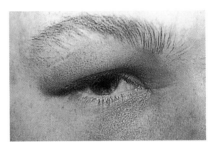

Inflammation of upper eyelid after expression of blackhead

*Allergy*
There may be a history of contact with an allergen, including animals, plants, chemicals, or cosmetics. Itching is an indicator of allergy. Treatment may include weak topical steroid ointment (hydrocortisone 1%) applied to the eyelid for a short period. The use of steroid ointments in the periorbital area should be monitored very closely, because of the potentially serious complications of even short term usage (glaucoma, cataract, herpes simplex keratitis, and atrophy of the skin).

*Herpes simplex*
This may present as a vesicular rash on the skin of the eyelid. There may be associated areas of vesicular eruption on the face. An "experienced" patient may be able to discern the prodromal tingling sensation. Early application of aciclovir cream will shorten the length and severity of the episode. Associated ocular herpetic disease should be considered if the eye is red, and the patient should then be referred immediately.

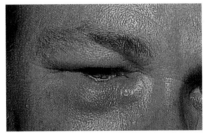

Dacryocystitis with associated lid inflammation

*Herpes zoster ophthalmicus (shingles)*
This presents as a vesicular rash over the distribution of the ophthalmic division of the fifth cranial nerve. There may be associated pain and the patient usually feels unwell.

The eye is often affected, particularly if the side of the nose is affected (which is innervated by a branch of the nasociliary nerve that also innervates the eye). Common ocular problems include conjunctivitis, keratitis, and uveitis. The eye is often shut because of oedema of the eyelid, but an attempt should be made to inspect the globe. If the eye is red or if there is visual disturbance the patient should be referred straight away. The ocular complications of herpes zoster may occur after the rash has resolved and even several months after primary infection, so the eye should be examined at each visit. Serious ophthalmic complications include glaucoma, cataract, uveitis, choroiditis, retinitis, and oculomotor palsies.

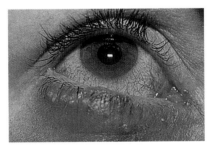

Herpes simplex with associated conjunctivitis

Treatment includes application of a wetting cream to the skin after crusting to prevent painful and disfiguring scars. If the eye is affected, topical antibiotics may prevent secondary infection, and aciclovir ointment is used. Oral antiviral therapy (for example, aciclovir) given early in the course of the disease may reduce the incidence of long term sequelae such as postherpetic neuralgia.

**Proptosis and enophthalmos**
Globe protrusion (proptosis) and sunken globe (enophthalmos) result in an asymmetrical position of the globes, which can often be best appreciated by standing behind

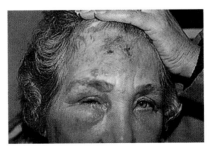

Herpes zoster ophthalmicus with swollen eyelids

the patient and looking from above their head (comparing the position of the eyes relative to the brows). The degree of proptosis or enophthalmos can be quantified by using an exophthalmometer. All patients with proptosis or enophthalmos need full ophthalmic and systemic investigation. There are many causes of proptosis and enophthalmos: some of the more common and important diseases are listed below.

### Causes of proptosis

*Orbital cellulitis*—**This is a potentially life threatening and blinding condition and must not be missed.** Orbital cellulitis usually results from the spread of infection from adjacent paranasal sinuses. It is particularly important in children, in whom blindness can ensue within hours, because the orbital walls are so thin. The patient usually presents with unilateral swollen eyelids that may or may not be red. Features to look for include:
- the patient is systemically unwell and febrile
- there is tenderness over the sinuses
- there is proptosis, chemosis, reduced vision, and restriction of eye movements.

The possibility of orbital cellulitis should always be kept in mind, especially in children, and patients should be referred immediately without any delay.

*Orbital inflammatory disease*—Non-specific orbital inflammatory disease can occur as an isolated finding or in association with a number of systemic vasculitides, including Wegener's granulomatosis.

*Thyroid eye disease*—See Chapter 12.

*Orbital lymphoma*—Deposits of lymphoma in the orbit need confirmation by orbital biopsy and should alert the clinician to the need for a full systemic work up for lymphoma elsewhere.

*Lacrimal gland tumour*—These tumours in the upper outer part of the orbit displace the globe inferiorly and medially.

*Orbital invasion from paranasal sinus infection or tumour*—Look for features of nasal or sinus disease in the history and examine the nose, oropharynx, and lymph nodes.

### Causes of enophthalmos

*Blowout orbital fracture*—See Chapter 5.

*Microphthalmos*—If one eye is smaller than the other due to developmental problems in embryogenesis, then the eye will appear enophthalmic. Microphthalmic eyes often have other problems including cataract and refractive errors.

*Cicatrising metastatic breast carcinoma*—This rare form of progressive enophthalmos is associated with very poor prognosis for survival.

## Malpositions of the eyelids and eyelashes

Malpositions of the eyelids and eyelashes are common and give rise to various symptoms, including irritation of the eye by lashes rubbing on it (entropion and ingrowing eyelashes) and watering of the eye caused by malposition of the punctum (ectropion).

The eyelids are folds of skin with fibrous plates in both the upper and lower lids, and the circular muscle (orbicularis) controls the closing of the eye. Any change in the muscles or supporting tissues may result in malposition of the lids.

### Entropion

Entropion is common, particularly in elderly patients with some spasm of the eyelids. The patient may present complaining of irritation caused by eyelashes rubbing on the cornea. This may

> **Orbital cellulitis can cause blindness if not treated immediately—particularly in children**

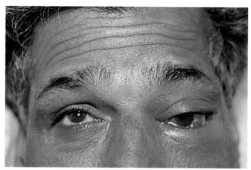

Orbital cellulitis: swollen eyelids, conjunctival swelling, displaced eyeball, and restricted eye movements

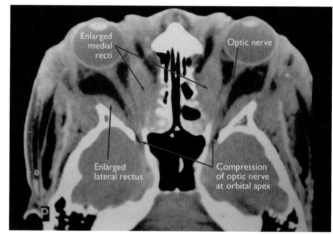

Computed tomogram of head/orbits showing enlarged extraocular muscles and optic nerve compression in thyroid eye disease

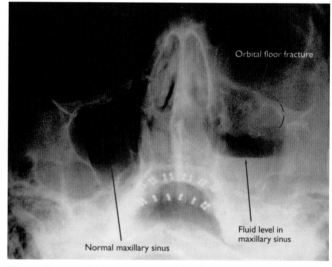

Blowout fracture of the orbit with fluid in the maxillary sinus

---

**Main symptoms of lid and lash malposition**
- Irritation of the eye by lashes rubbing on it (entropion)
- Watering of the eye caused by malposition of the punctum (ectropion)

be immediately apparent on examination but may be intermittent, in which case the lid may be in the normal position. The clue is that the eyelashes of the lower lid are pushed to the side by the regular inturning. The entropion can be brought on by asking the patient to close their eyes tightly, and then open them.

The great danger of entropion is ulceration and scarring of the cornea by the abrading eyelashes. The cornea should be examined by staining with fluorescein.

Temporary treatment of entropion consists of taping down the lower lid and applying chloramphenicol ointment. An operation under local anaesthesia is required to correct the entropion permanently. Scarring of the cornea, associated with entropion of the upper eyelid resulting from trachoma, is one of the most common causes of blindness worldwide.

### Trichiasis

Sometimes the lid may be in a normal position, but aberrant eyelashes may grow inwards. Trichiasis is more common in the presence of diseases of the eyelid such as blepharitis or trachoma. The eyelashes can be seen on examination, especially with magnification. They can be pulled out, but they frequently regrow.

The application of chloramphenicol ointment helps to prevent corneal damage, and electrolysis of the hair roots or cryotherapy may be necessary to stop the lashes regrowing.

### Ectropion

The initial complaint may be of a watery eye. The tears drain mainly via the lower punctum at the medial end of the lower lid. If the eyelid is not properly apposed to the eye, tears cannot flow into the punctum and the result is a watery eye.

The patient may also complain about the unsightly appearance of the ectropion. The most common reason for ectropion is laxity of tissues of the lid as a result of ageing, but it also occurs if the muscles are weak, as in the case of a facial nerve palsy. Scarring of the skin of the eyelid may also pull the lid margin down.

Ectropion can be rectified by an operation under local anaesthesia. Use of a simple lubricating ointment before the operation will help to protect the eye and prevent drying of the exposed conjunctiva.

### Ptosis

Ptosis or drooping of the eyelid may:

- *indicate a life threatening condition*—such as a third nerve palsy secondary to aneurysm or a Horner's syndrome secondary to carcinoma of the lung
- *indicate a disease that needs systemic treatment*—such as myasthenia gravis
- *cause irreversible amblyopia in a child* as a result of the lid obstructing vision. If there is any question of a ptosis obstructing vision in a child, he or she should be referred urgently.
- *be easily treated by a simple operation*—as in senile ptosis.

The patient will usually complain of a drooping eyelid. The upper eyelid is raised by the levator muscle, which is controlled by the third nerve. There is also Müller's muscle, which is controlled by the sympathetic nervous system. These muscles are attached to the fibrous plate in the eyelid and other lid structures. The ptosis can occur because of tissue defects, as described below.

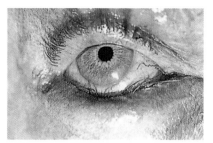

Entropion: inturning eyelashes may scratch and damage the cornea

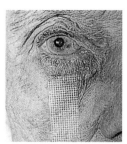

Temporary treatment of entropion

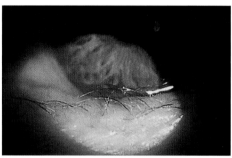

Trichiasis

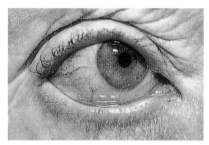

Ectropion with resulting epiphora

**Ptosis may occasionally:**
- Indicate a life threatening disease
- Indicate a systemic disease
- Cause amblyopia in children

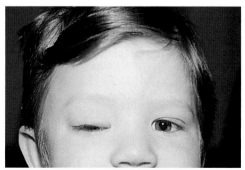

Ptosis caused by lid haemangioma; exclude amblyopia in a child

### Lid tissues

With ageing, the tissues of the eyelid become lax and the connections loosen, resulting in ptosis; this is common in the elderly. The eye movements and pupils should be normal. A pseudoptosis may occur when the skin of the upper lid sags and droops down over the lid margin. Both these conditions are amenable to relatively simple operations under local anaesthesia.

### Muscle tissue

It is important not to miss a general muscular disorder such as myasthenia gravis or dystrophia myotonica in a patient who presents with ptosis. Any diplopia, worsening symptoms throughout the day, and other muscular symptoms should lead one to suspect myasthenia. The patient's facies and a "clinging" handshake may give clues to the diagnosis of dystrophia myotonica.

### Nerve supply

A third nerve palsy may present as a ptosis. This, together with an abducted eye and dilated pupil, indicates the diagnosis. The patient should be referred urgently, as causes of third nerve palsy include a compressive lesion of the third nerve such as an aneurysm. Diabetes should be excluded.

### Horner's syndrome resulting from damage to the sympathetic chain

The pupil will be small but reactive, and sweating over the affected side of the face may be reduced. The eye movements should be normal. Causes of Horner's syndrome include lesions of the brain stem and spinal cord, dissection of the carotid artery and apical lung tumours, so the patient should be referred.

### Lid retraction

Lid retraction and associated lid lag are features of thyroid eye disease. These signs can occur in patients who are hyperthyroid, euthyroid, or hypothyroid.

### Blepharospasm

In essential blepharospasm there is episodic bilateral involuntary spasm of the orbicularis oculi muscles, which leads to unwanted forced closure of both eyes. Treatment options for this disabling condition include muscle relaxants, botulinum toxin injection, and surgical stripping of some of the orbicularis fibres.

## Lacrimal system

### Watering eye

Tears are produced by the lacrimal glands that lie in the upper lateral aspect of the orbits. They flow down across the eye along the lid margins and are spread across the eye by blinking. They then flow through the upper and lower puncta to the lacrimal sac and down the nasolacrimal duct into the nose.

Although rare, it is important to remember that children with congenital glaucoma may present with watery eyes. A watering eye may occur for several reasons.

### Excessive production of tears

This is rare, but can occur paradoxically in a patient with "dry eyes." Basal secretion of tears is inadequate and this results in drying of the eye. This gives rise to a reactive secretion of tears that causes epiphora. The patient may have a history of intermittent discomfort followed by watering of the eye.

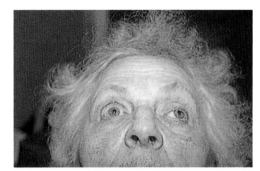

Left ptosis caused by pupil sparing third nerve palsy: note the divergent eye

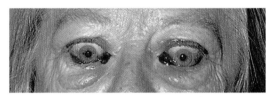

Clinical thyroid eye disease

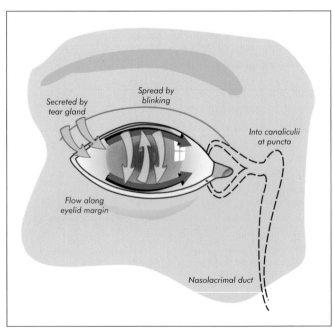

Secreted by tear gland

Spread by blinking

Into canaliculii at puncta

Flow along eyelid margin

Nasolacrimal duct

Normal tear flow

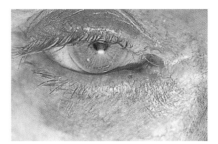

Watering eye caused by punctal ectropion

*Punctal malposition secondary to lid malposition*
The punctum must be well apposed to the eye to drain tears. Even mild ectropion can result in pooling of tears and overflow. Careful examination of the lid will usually show any malposition, which may be remedied by performing a minor operation.

*Punctal stenosis*
The punctum may close up and this will result in watering. If this is the case, the punctum cannot be seen easily on examination with a magnifying loupe. It can be surgically dilated or opened by a minor operation under local anaesthesia.

*Blockage of the lacrimal sac or nasolacrimal duct*
If the nasolacrimal duct is blocked and cannot be freed by syringing, an operation may be required. A common operation to bypass the obstruction is a dacryocystorhinostomy (DCR), in which a hole is made into the nose from the lacrimal sac. Sometimes plastic tubes are left in for several months to create a fistula. This major operation usually is performed under general anaesthesia.

A recent addition to the range of procedures for the surgical treatment of watery eyes is endoscopic DCR, in which the operation is performed through the nasal cavity. Good results are reported for this procedure, although external DCR still has the higher success rate.

In children the lacrimal drainage system may not be patent, particularly in the first few years of life. The child will present with a watering eye or sometimes with recurrent conjunctivitis. Treatment is usually with chloramphenicol eye drops for episodes of conjunctivitis, and the parents should massage the lacrimal sac daily to encourage flow. Most cases in childhood will resolve spontaneously. If the watering persists, the child may have to have the sac and duct syringed and probed under general anaesthesia. This procedure is generally best done between 12 and 24 months of age. If the blockage persists, a dacryocystorhinostomy may be performed when the child is older, but this is not often necessary.

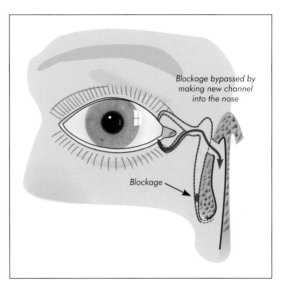

Blockage bypassed by making new channel into the nose

Blockage

Dacryocystorhinostomy

## Dry eye
Dry eye is common in the elderly, in whom tear secretion is reduced. The patient usually presents complaining of a chronic gritty sensation in the eye, which is not particularly red. Sjögren's syndrome is an autoimmune disease, with features of dry eyes and dry mouth, which can occur with certain connective tissue diseases such as rheumatoid arthritis. Drugs such as diuretics and agents with anticholinergic action (for example, certain drugs used in the treatment of depression, Parkinson's disease, and bladder instability) may also exacerbate the symptoms of dry eye.

Staining of the cornea may be apparent with fluorescein and rose bengal eye drops. (If rose bengal eye drops are used the eyes must be washed out very thoroughly, as these drops are a potent irritant.) A Schirmer's test can be carried out. A strip of filter paper is folded into the fornix and the advancing edge of tears is measured.

Treatment includes:

- *artificial tear drops*, which may be used as frequently as necessary (it may be necessary to use preservative free artificial tears in severe cases)
- *simple ointment*, which helps to give prolonged lubrication, particularly at night when tear secretion is minimal

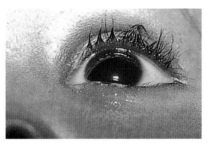

Blocked left nasolacrimal system in a child with recurrent discharge

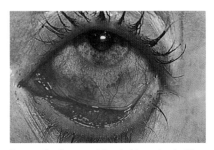

Dry eye in rheumatoid arthritis, stained with rose bengal drops, which stain damaged epithelium

27

- *acetylcysteine (mucolytic) eye drops*, which are useful if there is clumping of mucus on the eye (filamentary keratitis). However many patients find that the drops sting
- *treatment of any associated blepharitis*
- *temporary collagen or silicone lacrimal plugs* may be inserted into the upper or lower puncta, or both, to assess the effect of tear conservation
- *permanent punctal occlusion* can be produced by punctal cautery in refractory cases, often with dramatic effect.

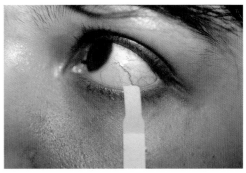

Schirmer's test

# 5 Injuries to the eye

An injury to the eye or its surrounding tissues is the most common cause for attendance at an eye hospital emergency department.

## History

The history of how the injury was sustained is crucial, as it gives clues as to what to look for during the examination. **If there is a history of any high velocity injury (particularly a hammer and chisel injury) or if glass was involved in the injury, then a penetrating injury must be strongly suspected and excluded.**

If there has been a forceful blunt injury (such as a punch), signs of a "blowout" fracture should be sought. The circumstances of the injury must be elicited and carefully recorded, as these may have important medicolegal implications. It may not be possible to get an accurate and reliable history from children if an injury is not witnessed by an adult. Such injuries should be treated with a high index of suspicion, as a penetrating eye injury may be present.

## Examination

A good examination is vital if there is a history of eye injury. Specific signs must be looked for or they will be missed. It is vital to test the visual acuity, both to establish a baseline value and to alert the examiner to the possibility of further problems. However, an acuity of 6/6 does not necessarily exclude serious problems—even a penetrating injury. The visual acuity may also have considerable medicolegal implications. Local anaesthetic may need to be used to obtain a good view, and fluorescein must be used to ensure no abrasions are missed.

## Corneal abrasions

Corneal abrasions are the most common result of blunt injury. They may follow injuries with foreign bodies, fingernails, or twigs. **Abrasions will be missed if fluorescein is not instilled.**

The aims of treatment are to ensure healing of the defect, prevent infection, and relieve pain.

Small abrasions can be treated with chloramphenicol ointment twice a day or eye drops four times a day until the eye has healed and symptoms are gone. Ointment blurs the vision more but provides longer lasting lubrication compared with eye drops. This will help prevent infection, lubricate the eye surface, and reduce discomfort.

For larger or more uncomfortable abrasions a double eye pad can be used with chloramphenicol ointment for a day or so until symptoms improve, or when the eye becomes uncomfortable with the pad (at which time it can be removed). The pad must be firm enough to keep the eyelid shut. Ointment or drops can then continue. If there is significant pain cycloplegic eye drops (cyclopentolate 1% or homatropine 2%) may help, although this will further blur the vision. Oral analgesia such as paracetamol or stronger non-steroidal anti-inflammatory drugs can also be used. Patients should be told to seek futher ophthalmological help if the eye continues to be painful, vision is blurred, or the eye develops a purulent discharge.

*Recurrent abrasions*—Occasionally the corneal epithelium may repeatedly break down where there has been a previous injury or there is an inherently weak adhesion between the epithelial cells and the basement membrane. These recurrences usually occur at night when there is little secretion

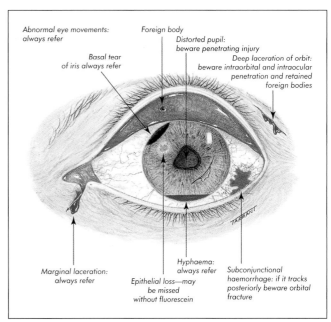

*Abnormal eye movements: always refer*

*Foreign body*

*Distorted pupil: beware penetrating injury*

*Basal tear of iris always refer*

*Deep laceration of orbit: beware intraorbital and intraocular penetration and retained foreign bodies*

*Marginal laceration: always refer*

*Epithelial loss—may be missed without fluorescein*

*Hyphaema: always refer*

*Subconjunctival haemorrhage: if it tracks posteriorly beware orbital fracture*

The injured eye

---

**Common types of eye injury**

- Corneal abrasions
- Foreign bodies
- Radiation damage
- Chemical damage
- Blunt injuries with hyphaema
- Penetrating injuries

---

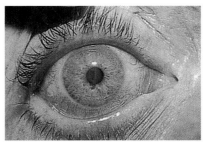

Corneal abrasion stained with fluorescein and illuminated with white light

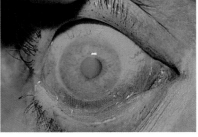

Corneal abrasion stained with fluorescein and illuminated with blue light

of tears and the epithelium may be torn off. Treatment is long term and entails drops during the day and ointment at night to lubricate the eye. Occasionally, a surgical procedure (such as epithelial debridement or corneal stromal puncture) may be carried out to enhance the adhesion between the epithelium and the underlying basement membrane.

## Foreign bodies

It is important to identify and remove conjunctival and corneal foreign bodies. A patient may not recall a foreign body having entered the eye, so it is essential to be on the lookout for a foreign body if a patient has an uncomfortable red eye. It may be necessary to use local anaesthetic both to examine the eye and to remove the foreign body. Although patients often request them, local anaesthetics should never be given to patients to use themselves, because they impede healing and further injury may occur to an anaesthetised eye.

Small loose conjunctival foreign bodies can be removed with the edge of a tissue or a cotton wool bud or they can be washed out with water. The upper lid must be everted to exclude a subtarsal foreign body, particularly if there are corneal scratches or a continuing feeling that a foreign body is present. However, this should not be done if a penetrating injury is suspected. Corneal foreign bodies are often more difficult to remove if they are metallic, because they are often "rusted on." They must be removed as they will prevent healing and rust may permanently stain the cornea. A cotton wool bud or the edge of a piece of cardboard can be used. If this does not work, a needle tip (or special rotary drill) can be used, but great care must be taken when using these as the eye may easily be damaged. If there is any doubt, these patients should be referred to an ophthalmologist. When the foreign body has been removed any remaining epithelial defect can be treated as an abrasion.

---

**Removal of a foreign body**

- Use local anaesthetic
- If the foreign body is loose, irrigate the eye
- If the foreign body is adherent, use a cotton wool bud or the edge of a piece of cardboard

---

## Radiation damage

The most common form of radiation damage occurs when welding has been carried out without adequate shielding of the eye. The corneal epithelium is damaged by the ultraviolet rays and the patient typically presents with painful, weeping eyes some hours after welding. (This condition is commonly known as "arc eye.")

Radiation damage can also occur after exposure to large amounts of reflected sunlight (for example, "snow blindness") or after ultraviolet light exposure in tanning machines. Treatment is as for a corneal abrasion.

## Chemical damage

**All chemical eye injuries are potentially blinding injuries**. If chemicals are splashed into the eye, the eye and the conjunctival sacs (fornices) should be washed out immediately with copious amounts of water. Acute management should consist of the three "Is": **Irrigate, Irrigate, Irrigate**. Alkalis are particularly damaging, and any loose bits such as lime should be removed from the conjunctival sac, with the aid of local

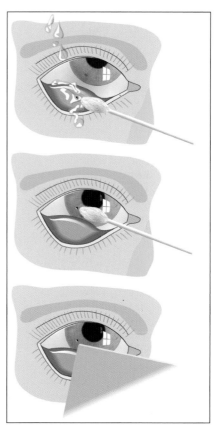

Removal of a foreign body from the eye

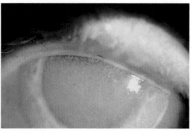

Lower lid gently pulled down to show a conjunctival foreign body. The cornea has also been perforated

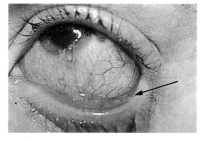

Subtarsal foreign body

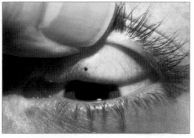

Cornea after welding damage, stained with fluorescein and illuminated with blue light

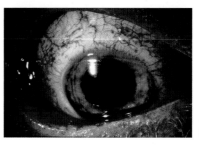

Chemical injury to the eye

anaesthetic if necessary. The patient should then be referred immediately to an ophthalmic department. If there is any doubt, irrigation should be continued for as long as possible with several litres of fluid.

# Blunt injuries

If a large object (such as a football) hits the eye most of the impact is usually taken by the orbital margin. If a smaller object (such as a squash ball) hits the area the eye itself may take most of the impact.

Haemorrhage may occur and a collection of blood may be plainly visible in the anterior chamber of the eye (hyphaema). Patients who sustain such injuries need to be reviewed at an eye unit as the pressure in the eye may rise, and further haemorrhages may require surgical intervention. Haemorrhage may also occur into the vitreous or in the retina, and this may be accompanied by a retinal detachment. All patients with visual impairment after blunt injury should be seen in an ophthalmic department.

The iris may also be damaged and the pupil may react poorly to light. This is particularly important in a patient with an associated head injury, as this may be interpreted as (or mask) the dilated pupil that is suggestive of an acute extradural haematoma. The lens may be damaged or dislocated and a cataract may develop. Damage to the drainage angle of the eye (which cannot be seen without a mirror contact lens and a slit lamp microscope) increases the chances of glaucoma developing in later life.

If the force of impact is transmitted to the orbit, an orbital fracture may occur (usually in the floor, which is thin and has little support). Clues to the presence of an inferior "blowout" fracture include diplopia, a recessed eye, defective eye movements (especially vertical), an ipsilateral nose bleed, and diminished sensation over the distribution of the infraorbital nerve. These patients need to be seen in an ophthalmic department for assessment and treatment of eye damage, and a maxillofacial department for repair of the orbital floor.

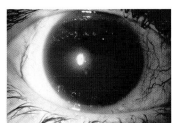

Hyphaema

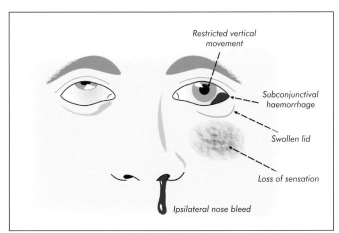

Signs of a left orbital blowout fracture (patient looking upwards)

**Dealing with chemical damage to the eye**
- Immediately wash out eye with water
- Remove loose particles
- Refer patient to ophthalmic department
- Beware alkalis

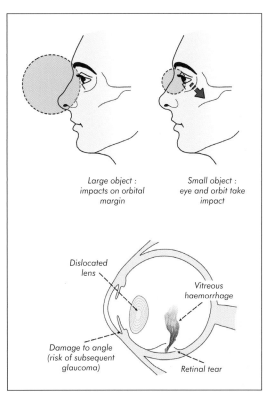

Complications of blunt trauma to the eye

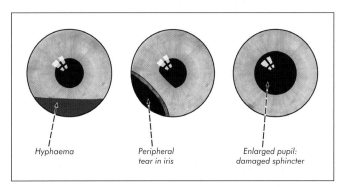

Signs of damage to the eye itself

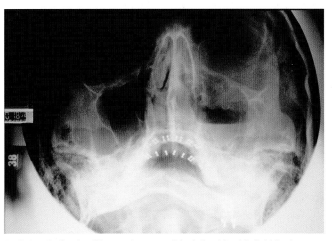

Radiograph showing blowout fracture of the left orbit with fluid in the maxillary sinus

# Penetrating injuries and eyelid lacerations

Lacerations of the eyelids need specialist attention if:

- *the lid margins have been torn*—these must be sewn together accurately
- *the lacrimal ducts have been damaged*—the laceration may involve the medial ends of the eyelids and it is likely that the lacrimal canaliculi will have been damaged, and these may need to be reapposed under the operating microscope
- *there is any suspicion of a foreign body or penetrating eyelid injury*—objects may easily penetrate the orbit and even the cranial cavity through the orbit.

Penetrating injuries of the eye can be missed because they may seal themselves, and the signs of abnormality are subtle. Any history of a high velocity injury (particularly a hammer and chisel injury) should lead one strongly to suspect a penetrating injury. In that case, the eye should be examined very gently and no pressure should be brought to bear on the globe. **It is possible to cause prolapse of intraocular contents and irreversible damage if the eye and orbit are not examined with great care.**

Signs to look for include a distorted pupil, cataract, prolapsed black uveal tissue on the ocular surface, and vitreous haemorrhage. The pupil should be dilated (if there is no head injury) and a thorough search made for an intraocular foreign body. If there is a suspicion of an intraocular or orbital foreign body then orbital *x* ray photographs, with the eye in up and down gaze, should be taken.

If the eye is clearly perforated it should be protected from any pressure by placing a shield over the eye, and the patient should be sent immediately to the nearest eye department.

Sympathetic ophthalmia, in which chronic inflammation develops in the normal fellow eye, is a potentially serious complication of any severe penetrating eye injury. The risk of this increases if a penetrating eye injury is left untreated. **All penetrating eye injuries should receive immediate specialist ophthalmic management without delay.**

**Penetrating eye injuries—beware:**
- Hammer and chisel
- Glass
- Knives
- Thorns
- Darts
- Pencils

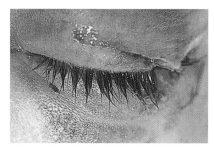

Lacerated eyelid

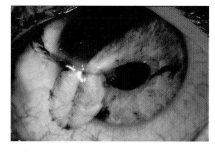

Penetrating eye injury

# 6 Acute visual disturbance

Acute disturbance of vision in a non-inflamed eye demands an accurate history, as the patient may have only just noticed a longstanding visual defect. Acute visual disturbance of unknown cause requires urgent referral.

## Symptoms and signs

In many cases the diagnosis can be made from the history. Symptoms of floaters or flashing lights suggest a vitreous detachment, a vitreous haemorrhage, or a retinal detachment. Horizontal field loss usually indicates a retinal vascular problem, whereas a vertical defect suggests a neuro-ophthalmic abnormality at or posterior to the optic chiasm. If there is central field loss ("I can't see things in the centre of my vision" or "I can't see people's faces") there may be a disorder at the macula or within the optic nerve. Associated **systemic** symptoms should be elicited. Severe headache and jaw claudication in an older person may suggest giant cell arteritis. A previous history of migraine, diabetes mellitus, cerebrovascular disease, valvular heart disease, carotid artery disease, or multiple sclerosis may give clues to the underlying aetiology of the acute visual loss. It is important to take a careful history regarding the onset of acute visual loss, as a patient may sometimes only notice that one eye has (longstanding) reduced vision when they inadvertently cover the good eye.

The visual acuity gives a strong clue to the diagnosis. Poor visual acuity such as count fingers (CF), hand movements (HM), perception of light only (PL) or no perception of light (NPL) suggest a severe insult to the retina or optic nerve (for example, a vascular occlusive event).

---

**History and examination of a patient with acute visual disturbance**

**History**
- Floaters
- Field loss
- Zigzag lines
- Flashing lights
- Headache
- Pain on moving eye

**Examination**
- Acuity
- Pupil reactions
- Appearance of retina, macula, and optic nerve
- Red reflex
- Field loss

---

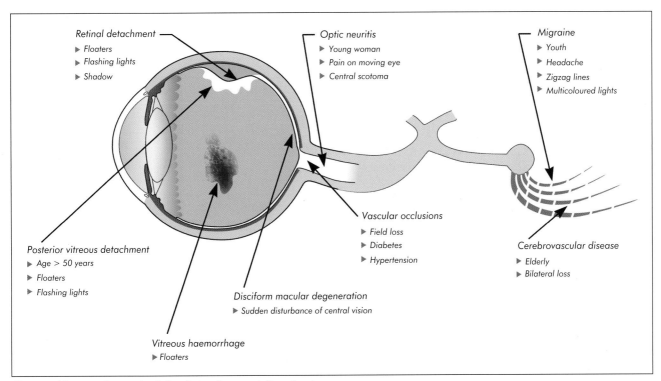

Causes and features of acute visual disturbance (in a non-inflamed eye)

Obstruction of the red reflex on ophthalmoscopy suggests a vitreous haemorrhage, although the patient may have a pre-existing cataract. The appearance of the macula, remaining retina, and head of the optic nerve will indicate the diagnosis if there has been haemorrhage or arterial or venous occlusion in these areas.

If there is any uncertainty about the cause of acute visual loss, then the patient should be referred to an eye specialist immediately. Many of the causes are treatable if detected at an early stage.

## Posterior vitreous detachment

Posterior vitreous detachment is the most common cause of the acute onset of floaters, particularly with advancing age, and is one of the most common causes of acute visual disturbance.

*History*—The patient presents complaining of floaters. In posterior vitreous detachment, the vitreous body collapses and detaches from the retina. If there are associated flashing lights it suggests that there may be traction on the retina, which may result in a retinal hole and a subsequent retinal detachment.

*Examination*—The visual acuity is characteristically normal, and there should be no loss of visual field.

*Management*—Patients with an acute posterior vitreous detachment should have an urgent (same day) ophthalmic assessment, so that any retinal breaks or detachment can be identified and treated at an early stage. The patient may require a further visit one to two months later to exclude subsequent development of a retinal hole.

## Vitreous haemorrhage

*History*—The patient complains of a sudden onset of floaters, or "blobs," in the vision. The visual acuity may be normal or, if the haemorrhage is dense, it may be reduced. Flashing lights indicate retinal traction and are a dangerous symptom. Haemorrhage may occur from spontaneous rupture of vessels, avulsion of vessels during retinal traction, or bleeding from abnormal new vessels. If the patient is shortsighted, retinal detachment is more likely. If there is associated diabetes mellitus the patient may have bled from new vessels and the vitreous haemorrhage may herald potentially sight threatening diabetic retinopathy.

*Examination*—The visual acuity depends on the extent of the haemorrhage. Projection of light is accurate unless the haemorrhage is extremely dense. Ophthalmoscopy shows the red reflex to be reduced; there may be clots of blood that move with the vitreous.

*Management*—The patient should be referred to an ophthalmologist to exclude a retinal detachment. Ultrasound examination of the eye may be useful, particularly if the haemorrhage precludes a view of the retina. Underlying causes such as diabetes must also be excluded. If a vitreous haemorrhage fails to clear spontaneously the patient may benefit from having the vitreous removed (vitrectomy).

## Retinal detachment

Retinal detachment should be suspected from the history. It is only when the detachment is advanced that the vision and the visual fields are affected and the detachment becomes readily visible on direct ophthalmoscopy.

*History*—The patient may complain of a sudden onset of floaters, indicating pigment or blood in the vitreous, and

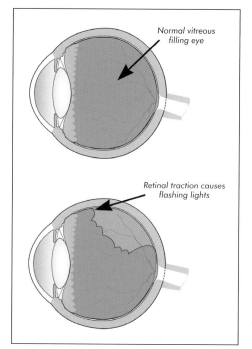

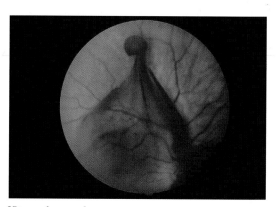

*Normal vitreous filling eye*

*Retinal traction causes flashing lights*

Posterior vitreous detachment causing retinal traction and a "flashing lights" sensation

Vitreous haemorrhage

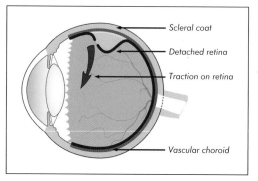

Scleral coat

Detached retina

Traction on retina

Vascular choroid

Retinal detachment. Only visible on direct ophthalmoscopy when detachment is advanced

flashing lights caused by traction on the retina. These, however, are not invariable and the patient may not present until there is field loss when the area of detachment is sufficiently large or a deterioration in visual acuity if the macula is detached. Retinal detachment is more likely to occur if the retina is thin (in the shortsighted patient) or damaged (by trauma) or if the ocular dynamics have been disturbed (by a previous cataract operation). Traction from a contracting membrane after vitreous haemorrhage in a patient with diabetes can also cause a retinal detachment.

*Examination*—Visual acuity is normal if the macula is still attached, but the acuity is reduced to counting fingers or hand movements if the macula is detached. Field loss (not complete in the early stages) is dependent on the size and location of the detachment. Direct ophthalmoscopy will not detect the abnormality if the detachment is small; detached retinal folds may be seen in larger detachments.

*Management*—The patient should be referred urgently. Only small retinal holes with no associated fluid under the retina can be treated with a laser, which causes an inflammatory reaction that seals the hole. True detachments usually require an operation to seal any holes, reduce vitreous traction, and if necessary drain fluid from beneath the neuroretina. A vitrectomy may be required, which is carried out using fine microsurgical cutting instruments inserted into the eye with fibreoptic illumination. This may be combined with the use of special intraocular gases (for example, sulphur hexafluoride) or silicone oil to keep the retina flat. If gas is used the patient may have to posture face down for several weeks after surgery in cases of retinal detachment, and must not travel by air (the intraocular gas expands at altitude) until most of the gas in the eye has been absorbed.

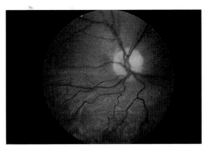

Detached retinal folds—inferior detachment

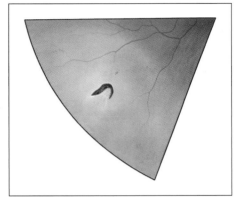

Retinal tear

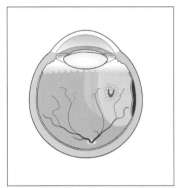

Cryotherapy is used to treat the retinal hole causing the retinal detachment

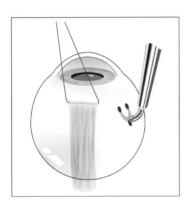

Cryotherapy (freezing treatment) is applied to the sclera overlying the retinal tear

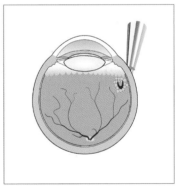

Cryotherapy causes scarring, which seals the retinal hole

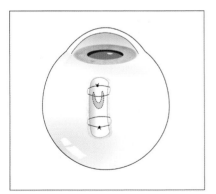

A piece of silicone is stitched to the scleral surface causing indentation, which closes the retinal hole and relieves vitreous traction

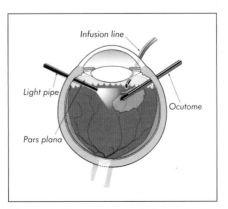

Microsurgical instruments can be inserted inside the eye to remove the vitreous gel in complicated retinal detachment surgery

# Arterial occlusion

*History*—The patient complains of a sudden onset of visual disturbance, often described as a "greyout" of the vision or as a "curtain" descending over the vision, in one or both eyes. This may be temporary (amaurosis fugax) if the obstruction dislodges or permanent if tissue infarction occurs.

*Examination*—In retinal artery occlusion the visual acuity depends on whether the macula or its fibres are affected. There may be no direct pupillary reaction if there is a complete occlusion with a dense relative afferent pupil defect. The extent of visual field loss depends on the area of retina affected. The retinal artery and its branches supply the inner two thirds of the neuroretina, and the outer third is supplied by the choroid. The arteries may be blocked by atherosclerosis, thrombosis, or emboli, and the attacks may be associated with a history of transient ischaemic attacks if the aetiology is embolic. When the retina infarcts it becomes oedematous and pale and masks the choroidal circulation except at the macula, which is extremely thin—hence the "cherry red spot" appearance.

Ophthalmoscopy may be normal initially, before oedema is established, and indeed the retinal appearance may return to normal after the oedema resolves. Plaques of cholesterol or calcium occasionally may be seen in the vessels. In posterior ciliary artery occlusion there is infarction of the optic nerve head, which has a pale swollen appearance with peripapillary haemorrhage. This appearance may be mistaken for papilloedema. Papilloedema, however, is usually bilateral and the visual acuity is not affected until late in its development.

## Two main arterial systems that may occlude in the posterior segment of the eye

- Central or branch retinal arteries—occlusion leads to retinal infarction
- Posterior ciliary arteries—occlusion leads to optic nerve head infarction (arteritic and non-arteritic anterior ischaemic optic neuropathy)

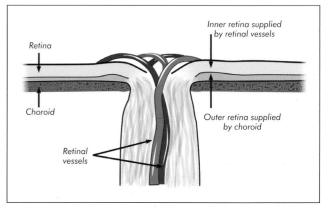

Blood supply of retina

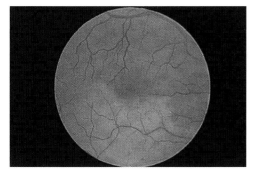

Arterial occlusion—infarction of lower half of retina

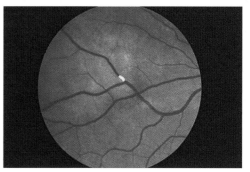

Arterial occlusion—embolus

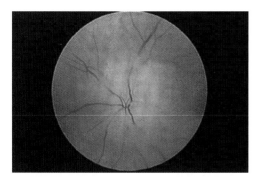

Arterial occlusion—ischaemic optic nerve head pale and swollen

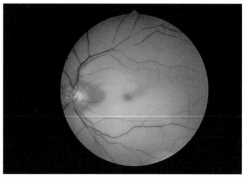

Central retinal artery occlusion (CRAO) and cherry red spot at the macula

*Management*—**Giant cell arteritis** must be excluded by the history and examination, and by checking the erythrocyte sedimentation rate. Rapid onset of second eye involvement can occur in giant cell arteritis and this condition is an ophthalmic and medical emergency. Immediate high dose intravenous steroid therapy is indicated. Emboli from the carotid arteries and heart should be excluded. Attempts may be made to open up the arterial circulation in acute cases by ocular massage, rapid reduction in intraocular pressure medically, anterior chamber paracentesis, or by carbon dioxide rebreathing to cause arterial dilatation. Factors predisposing to vascular disease (for example, smoking, diabetes, and hyperlipidaemia) should be identified and dealt with.

# Venous occlusion

*History*—The visual acuity will be disturbed only if the occlusion affects the temporal vascular arcades and damages the macula. Patients may otherwise complain only of a vague visual disturbance or of field loss. The arteries and veins share a common sheath in the eye, and venous occlusion most commonly occurs where arteries and veins cross, and in the head of the nerve. Thus raised arterial pressure can give rise to venous occlusion. Hyperviscosity (for example, in myeloma) and increased "stickiness" of the blood (as in diabetes mellitus) will also predispose to venous occlusion. This leads to haemorrhages and oedema of the retina. Occlusion of the central retinal vein within the head of the nerve leads to swelling of the optic disc.

*Examination*—Visual acuity will not be affected unless the macula is damaged. There may be some peripheral field loss if a branch occlusion has occurred. Ophthalmoscopy shows characteristic flame haemorrhages in the affected areas, with a swollen disc if there is occlusion of the central vein. An afferent pupillary defect and retinal cotton wool spots imply an ischaemic, damaged retina and are a bad prognostic sign.

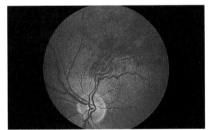

Branch retinal vein occlusion

*Management*—Hypertension, diabetes mellitus, hyperviscosity syndromes, and chronic glaucoma must be identified and treated if present. It is important to consider systemic investigation for inherited and acquired coagulopathies in young patients with retinal venous occlusive disease. Antiplatelet therapy should be considered if there are no contraindications. There is evidence that involvement of a physician in the care of patients with retinal occlusive disease can reduce the chance of second eye involvement and serious systemic vascular disease.

If the retina becomes ischaemic it stimulates the formation of new vessels on the iris (rubeosis) and subsequent neovascularisation of the angle may lead to secondary glaucoma. This may occur several months after the initial venous occlusion. Such rubeotic glaucoma is a serious condition and has the potential to render the eye both blind and painful. Fluorescein angiography may be useful. This involves the injection of intravenous fluorescein and sequential

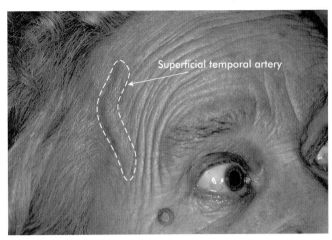

Temporal arteritis

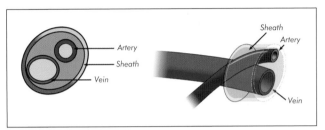

Raised blood pressure causes thickening of the arteries, which leads to compression of veins

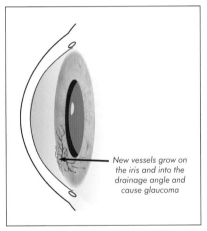

New vessels grow on the iris and into the drainage angle and cause glaucoma

Neovascularisation of the iris induced by vasoproliferative factors released from the ischaemic retina

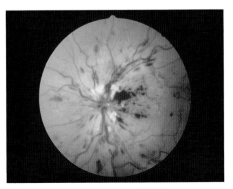

Central retinal vein occlusion (CRVO)

fundus photography with light filters to identify areas of poor perfusion and fluorescein leakage. Laser treatment is used to ablate the ischaemic retina in an attempt to prevent new vessel formation.

## Disciform macular degeneration

*History*—The patient notices a sudden disturbance of central vision. Straight lines may seem wavy and objects may be distorted, even seeming larger or smaller than normal. Eventually, central vision may be lost completely. This central area of visual distortion or loss moves as the patient tries to look around it. The layer under the neuro retina is the black retinal pigment epithelium. Most commonly with increasing age (the patient is normally over 60) and in certain conditions (for example, high myopia) neovascular membranes may develop under this layer in the macular region. These membranes may leak fluid or bleed and cause an acute disturbance of vision.

*Examination*—Visual acuity depends on the extent of macular involvement. If the patient looks at a grid pattern (Amsler chart) the lines may seem distorted in the central area, although the peripheral fields are normal. On fundal examination the macula may look normal or there may be a raised area within it. Haemorrhage in the retina is red but it appears black if it is under the retinal pigment epithelium. There may be associated deposits of yellow degenerative retinal products (drusen).

*Management*—Some cases are treatable with a laser that occludes these neovascular membranes. The abnormal areas of leaking blood vessels are identified by the use of intravenous dye injection in combination with fundus photography (fluorescein angiography and indocyanine green angiography). A patient who has had a subretinal neovascular membrane in one eye that has destroyed central vision is at risk of the same thing occurring in the other eye. The problem with laser treatment is that it may cause immediate worsening of vision, with benefit only in the long term. Trials are still underway to determine the role of radiation therapy in preventing the progression of the neovascular membranes. A recent development in the treatment of choroidal neovascularisation is the use of photodynamic therapy (PDT). This technique is described in Chapter 10.

## Optic or retrobulbar neuritis

*History*—The patient is usually a woman aged between 20 and 40, who complains of a disturbance of vision of one eye. There is usually pain that worsens on movement of the eye. There may have been previous attacks.

*Examination*—The visual acuity may range from 6/6 to perception of light. Despite a "normal" visual acuity, the patient usually has an afferent pupillary defect and may notice that the colour red looks faded when viewed with the affected eye (red desaturation). The field defect is usually a central field loss (central scotoma). It is extremely important to test the field of the other eye, as a field defect in the "good" eye may suggest a lesion of the optic chiasm or tract (for example, a pituitary adenoma). If the "inflammation" is anterior in the nerve, the optic disc will be swollen. Accompanying symptoms of general demyelinating disease such as pins and needles, weakness, and incontinence suggest multiple sclerosis.

*Management*—Most patients recover spontaneously, but they may be left with diminished acuity and optic atrophy. Treatment with systemic steroids does not alter the long term visual prognosis but may hasten recovery. Systemic steroids may, in selected patients, reduce the incidence of subsequent

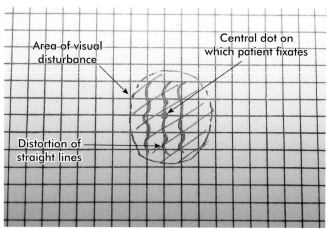

Amsler chart: distortion seen by patient with age-related macular degeneration

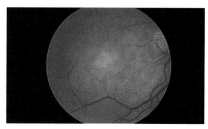

Leakage of fluid at macula (right eye)

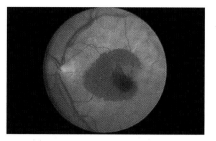

Macular haemorrhage (left eye)

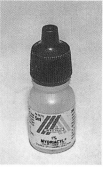

Red as seen by normal eye

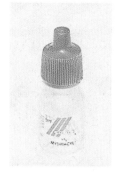

Red desaturation

**Treatment with steroids does not alter the visual prognosis, but it may hasten recovery in retrobulbar neuritis**

multiple sclerosis. Referral to a neurologist is necessary. Debate continues regarding the use of systemic steroids and other disease modifying agents such as β interferon. If there is doubt about the diagnosis, with atypical clinical features or history, then the patient may need further investigation to exclude a space occupying lesion.

# Cardiovascular and cerebrovascular disease

*History*—Intermittent episodes of transient visual loss (amaurosis fugax) and bilateral permanent visual field loss may be caused by either cardiovascular or cerebrovascular disease. The characteristic feature of a posterior visual pathway lesion is a homonymous nature to the hemianopic or quadrantanopic visual field defect, which respects the vertical midline. The patient may have a hemiparesis or hemisensory disturbance on the same side as the visual field loss. Patients sometimes complain of "the beginning or end of a line of print disappearing," and some may complain of a decrease in acuity.

The visual pathways pass through a large area of the cerebral hemispheres, and any vascular occlusion in these areas will affect these pathways. This is in contrast to vascular lesions in the eye or optic nerve, which either affect the whole field of one eye or if partial tend to respect the horizontal meridian in that eye. More posteriorly placed lesions in the brain tend to spare the macular vision in the affected fields.

*Examination*—The visual acuity should be preserved, although patients may say half (either the left or right hand side) of the Snellen chart is missing.

*Management*—It is important to make the diagnosis and exclude any underlying cause for the visual pathway damage. The following conditions should be excluded:

- Hypertension
- Diabetes mellitus
- Abnormal serum lipid profile
- Hyperviscosity syndromes
- Cardiac arrhythmias
- Cardiac embolic disease
- Carotid artery disease
- Giant cell arteritis.

The visual field defects sometimes improve with time, and patients should be taught to compensate for their field defect with appropriate head and eye movements. These techniques can be taught in low vision assessment clinics.

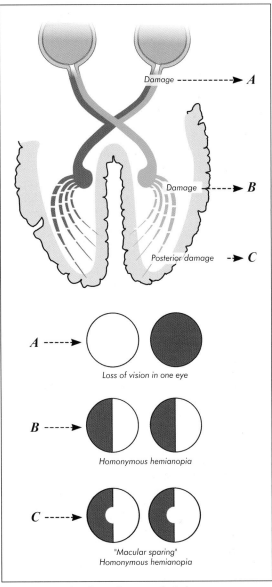

Damage to visual pathways from vascular lesions

# Migraine

*History*—Migraine may present initially with symptoms of visual loss. The features are well known and include:

- *a family history of migraine*
- *attacks set off by certain stimuli*—for example, particular foods
- *fortification spectra in both eyes*—these include zigzag lines and multicoloured flashes of light
- *associated headache and nausea*—although these symptoms may not be present.

**However, if patients present for the first time after 40 years of age with migraine and associated neurological symptoms or signs, consider the need for further investigation.**

*Examination*—The patient may have a bilateral field defect but this usually resolves within a few hours.

*Management*—Conventional treatment with analgesics and antiemetics may be necessary. Long term prophylaxis may be required if attacks occur often.

---

**Migraine—particular visual features**
- Zigzag lines
- Multicoloured flashing lights

---

# 7   Gradual visual disturbance, partial sight, and "blindness"

## Causes of gradual visual loss

### Refractive errors

The pinhole test is a most useful test for identifying refractive errors. If there is a refractive error, the vision will improve when the pinhole is used. A patient with thick glasses should wear them for the pinhole test. Once other causes of visual loss have been excluded, the patient can be sent to an optometrist for refraction and correction of refractive error (for example, glasses).

### Corneal disease

Various disorders can cause gradual loss of the corneal endothelial cells and increasing oedema of the cornea (for example, Fuch's endothelial dystrophy). This leads to a gradual decrease in visual acuity that does not improve substantially with a pinhole. If the damage is advanced the cornea may appear opaque. A corneal graft from a donor may be required.

### Cataract

This is probably the most common cause of gradual visual loss. It can be diagnosed through testing the red reflex. The patient should be referred if the visual disturbance interferes appreciably with their lifestyle. If a patient with a cataract cannot project light or has an afferent pupillary defect, however, other diseases such as a retinal detachment must be excluded.

### Primary open angle glaucoma

Unfortunately, the patient may not complain of visual disturbance until late in the course of the disease; hence the need for screening. Primary open angle glaucoma should, however, be excluded in any patient complaining of gradual visual loss. Establish whether there is any family history of glaucoma. The vision may still be 6/6, so the visual field should be checked with a red pin. Also check for cupping of, or asymmetry between, the optic discs.

### Age-related macular degeneration

This may occur gradually and is typified by loss of the central field. There are usually pigmentary changes at the macula. The disease occurs in both eyes, but it may be asymmetrical, and it is more common in shortsighted people. The gradual deterioration is not treatable, but if acute visual distortion develops this may indicate a leaking area under the retina (choroidal neovascularisation), which may respond to laser photocoagulation or photodynamic therapy.

### Macular hole

A macular hole is a full thickness absence of neural tissue at the centre of the macula. Between 10 and 20% of full thickness macular holes (FTMH) will become bilateral. Patients usually present with painless loss of central vision or distortion of the central visual field, although early macular holes may be asymptomatic. Patients with established FTMH can be treated with vitrectomy and instillation of intraocular gas (to provide retinal tamponade), which have a high chance of closing the hole successfully.

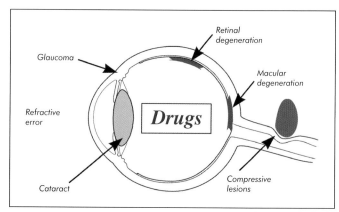

Causes of gradual visual loss

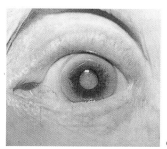

Cataract

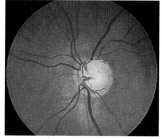

Glaucomatous cupping of the optic disc

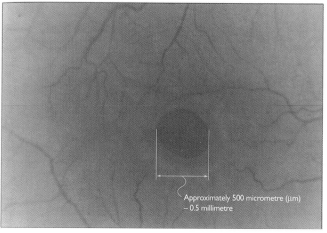

Macular hole

### Diabetic maculopathy

Diabetic retinopathy occurs in both insulin dependent and non-insulin dependent diabetics and affects all age groups. The patient may or may not give a history of diabetes, although the longer the duration of the diabetes, the more likely the patient is to have retinopathy. Remember that although the patient may describe the onset of visual loss as gradual, sight threatening diabetic retinopathy may still be present.

Non-proliferative diabetic retinopathy is typified by microaneurysms, dot haemorrhages, and hard yellow exudates with well defined edges. There also may be oedema of the macula, which is less easily identified but can lead to a fall in visual acuity. Non-proliferative diabetic retinopathy at the macula (diabetic maculopathy) is the major cause of blindness in maturity onset (type 2) diabetes, but it also occurs in younger, insulin dependent (type 1) diabetic patients. Some forms of diabetic maculopathy may be amenable to focal laser photocoagulation. Proliferative retinopathy, typified by the presence of new vessels, requires urgent referral for treatment.

### Hereditary degeneration of the retina

These conditions are relatively rare (for example, retinitis pigmentosa) but should be suspected if there is a family history of visual deterioration. Symptoms include night blindness and intolerance to light. Most types of retinal degeneration are not yet treatable, but some are associated with metabolic disorders that can be treated. These patients need to be referred to an ophthalmologist, preferably with a special interest in these conditions, for diagnosis and any possible treatments.

Patients with severe visual impairment may develop visual hallucinations and sleep disturbance. It is particularly important for these patients to have an opportunity to discuss their diagnosis and prognosis and to have genetic counselling. Patients can be helped through psychosocial counselling (see below, Management of gradual visual loss).

### Compressive lesions of the optic pathways

These are relatively rare, but should always be considered. Clues in the history and examination include headaches, focal neurological signs, or endocrinological abnormalities such as acromegaly. There should not be an afferent pupillary defect in most patients with cataract, macular degeneration, or refractive error. Therefore if an afferent defect is seen, suspect a compressive or other lesion of the optic pathways. Testing of the visual fields may show a bitemporal field defect due to a pituitary tumour. The optic discs should be checked for optic atrophy and papilloedema.

### Drugs

Several drugs may cause gradual visual loss. In particular, a history of excessive alcohol intake or smoking; methanol ingestion; or the taking of chloroquine, hydroxychloroquine, isoniazid, thioridazine, isotretinoin, tetracycline, or ethambutol should lead to the suspicion of drug induced visual deterioration. Systemic, inhaled, or topical corticosteroids may cause cataracts and glaucoma.

## Management of gradual visual loss

The initial management of gradual visual loss depends on the cause. Refractive errors usually require no more than a pair of glasses. Cataracts can be removed and an artificial lens implanted. Glaucoma requires treatment to lower the intraocular pressure.

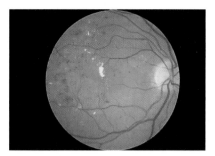
Background retinopathy with macular changes and good vision: refer

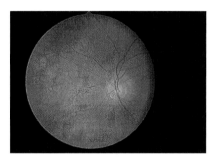
Retinitis pigmentosa: pigmentation and attenuated vessels

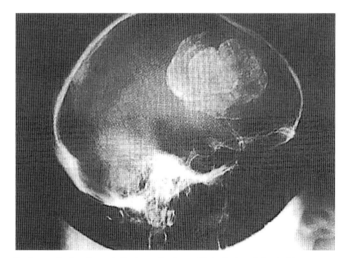
Radiograph showing calcified meningioma. Note that a plain skull radiograph will not show most intracranial tumours

**Patients with unexplained visual loss always should be referred**

However, a substantial number of conditions are not amenable to medical or surgical treatment. Despite this, there is still much that the patient can do. Local authority services and a large number of voluntary organisations offer practical help and support.

## Maximising low vision

Many eye departments have a low vision aids service, usually run by an optometrist, which may offer such aids on loan.

### Good lighting

The patient should use adequate lighting; a brighter light bulb may make all the difference. For reading, patients should have a strong light placed behind them. This reduces glare, maximises contrast between the print and the page, and may reduce excessive pupillary constriction that would otherwise impair vision, especially if the patient has cataracts. A helpful booklet, *Lighting and low vision*, is available from the Partially Sighted Society.

### Magnifying aids

A simple magnifying glass may be a great help. There are also special magnifying aids that can be attached to the patient's glasses. Unlike a simple magnifying glass, these magnify the print without the patient having to get extremely close to it. Closed circuit television can be used to magnify text.

### Large print

Most public libraries stock large print books. Many official forms and documents are now available in large print format.

### Closed circuit television

Books can be placed under the camera and magnified with the zoom lens. They are then viewed on the television screen. Grants can be obtained to help with the purchase of these units.

### Home aids

There is a wide range of aids for the home, available through local voluntary groups and the Royal National Institute for the Blind (RNIB). For tactile markings for cookers, contact the local electricity and gas suppliers.

## Psychosocial support

The diagnosis of a disease that causes substantial visual disability can be devastating for patients, particularly for the parents of children with these conditions. Psychosocial support is needed following the diagnosis of a serious eye condition and at subsequent stages of sight loss. Some specialised eye departments provide this help as part of a multidisciplinary team. However, the vast majority of patients only receive this help via their local authority social services department or a voluntary society for the visually impaired.

A summary of guidelines, and more detailed guidelines for professionals involved with newly diagnosed blind and partially sighted children and their families, can be obtained free from the RNIB.

### Self help support groups and other organisations

Visually impaired people and their families need advice, practical help, and information, both at the time of diagnosis and at subsequent stages of sight loss. These can be provided by support groups and other organisations.

### Genetic counselling

Patients with hereditary visual problems should have the opportunity to discuss the implications with a geneticist.

---

**Aids to maximise low vision**
- Strong light from behind for reading
- Magnifying aids
- Large print books
- Closed circuit television
- Home aids

---

**Helpful organisations**

**Action for Blind People**
14-16 Verney Road, London SE16 3DZ
Tel: 020 7635 4800
email: info@afbp.org
Website: www.afbp.org (accessed 28 Nov 2003)
Provides information and advisory service for visually impaired people, including benefits, grants, and employment

**Albinism Fellowship**
PO Box 77, Nr Burnley, Lancashire BB11 5GN
Tel: 01282 771900 (helpline open Tues and Fri 2-3pm)
email: albinism@bughunter.co.uk
Website: www.albinism.org.uk (accessed 28 Nov 2003)
Support and information for anyone with the eye condition albinism

**Association of Blind Asians (ABA)**
Garrow House, 190 Kensal Road
North Kensington, London W10 5BN
Tel: 020 8962 2633
email: bhartipunjani@hotmail.com or abaoffice@aol.com
Working for the welfare of visually impaired Asian people and their families, providing information, advice, and support

**Benefits Agency Helpline**
Tel: 0800 882200 (freephone)
Website: www.dwp.gov.uk (accessed 28 Nov 2003)
Advice on benefits

**British Retinitis Pigmentosa Society**
PO Box 350, Buckingham MK18 1GZ
Helpline: 01280 860363 (Mon-Fri 9.30-5.00 and 6.00-9.30pm)
Tel: 01280 821334
email: info@brps.org.uk
Website: www.brps.org.uk (accessed 28 Nov 2003)
Specialist support group for people with retinitis pigmentosa

**Contact a Family**
209-211 City Road, London EC1V 1JN
Helpline: 0808 808 3555 (freephone)
email: info@cafamily.org.uk
Website: www.cafamily.org.uk (accessed 28 Nov 2003)
National organisation that links up families with specialist support groups. Advice on setting up a local support group. Publications and information

**Disability Law Service**
39-45 Cavell Street, London E1 2BP
Tel: 020 7791 9800
email: advice@dis.org.uk
Provides legal advice and representation for disabled people on community care, benefits, consumer and contract law, disability discrimination, education, and employment

Most regions have a genetic counselling service. Some specialist eye hospitals have genetic counsellors in the multidisciplinary team.

## Registration as partially sighted or blind

Blind or partially sighted registration is not essential, but it helps patients to access financial benefits and specialist support and advice from local authorities. Once the local authority social service department has received the registration form, a number of support services should then be available to the visually impaired person. Each local authority keeps a register of blind and partially sighted people living within the area. The social worker is the key person to contact, but a visually impaired person may need a range of support services.

The patient should be referred to a consultant ophthalmologist who, with the patient's agreement, completes form BD8 (or BP1 for Scotland). The requirements for registration are described below.

*Partially sighted*—The patient must have vision of 6/60 or worse in both eyes. The vision can be better than 6/60 if the visual fields are markedly reduced; for example, a patient with 6/6 vision but severely restricted fields caused by primary open angle glaucoma. A patient who has an homonymous hemianopia following a stroke should be offered the option of being registered partially sighted.

*Blind*—The current statutory definition of blindness is "that a person should be so blind as to be unable to perform any work for which eyesight is essential." However, many registered blind people continue in their employment with appropriate resources. The guidelines for registration as blind are a visual acuity of 3/60 or worse in both eyes. Again, the visual acuity can be better than this if the visual fields are abnormal.

These criteria are flexible and the final decision is left to the consultant ophthalmologist, who will take other ocular problems into consideration. It is important that the patient does not feel that all hope is lost and that eventually everything will go completely "dark." In particular, for patients with age-related macular degeneration, only the central vision is lost. In this case patients can be told that they will not go blind because they will still have peripheral vision. A patient with vision of counting fingers still may be virtually independent within the home, despite being registered as blind.

## Special education and training

Most visually impaired children attend mainstream schools with specialist support. For some children it may be appropriate to attend a specialist school for the visually impaired. The local education authority's sensory impairment team will assess the needs of each child. Further help and advice for parents, particularly about their child's placement and their right of appeal, is offered by the RNIB.

## Employment and training

Information and advice is available from the RNIB Employment Network, the Disability Employment Adviser at the local job centre (employment services), Action for Blind People, and the Royal London Society for the Blind. Practical support, such as modifications to equipment and help with fares to and from work, can be accessed through the Disability Employment Adviser at the local job centre.

## Mobility and technical training

Rehabilitation officers employed by local authorities teach a whole range of skills, such as Braille, mobility skills, and daily living skills. In some areas this work is undertaken by staff from

**Helpful organisations (continued)**

**Guide Dogs for the Blind Association**
Hillfields, Burghfield Common
Reading, Berkshire RG7 3YG
Tel: 0870 600 2323
email: guidedogs@guidedogs.org.uk
Website: www.guidedogs.org.uk (accessed 28 Nov 2003)
Provides guide dogs for partially sighted and blind people, plus long cane training and rehabilitation for daily living

**International Glaucoma Association (see also "Tadpoles Parent Support Group")**
108C Warner Road, London SE5 9HQ
Tel: 020 7737 3265
email: info@iga.org.uk
Website: www.iga.org.uk (accessed 28 Nov 2003)
Information, support, and practical advice for people living with glaucoma and the professionals who work with them

**LOOK (National Federation of Families with Visually Impaired Children)**
c/o Queen Alexandra College, 49 Court Oak Road
Harborne, Birmingham B17 9TG
Tel: 0121 428 5038
email: office@look-uk.org
Website: www.look-uk.org (accessed 28 Nov 2003)
Provides practical help, support, advice, information, and local contacts, through local parent support groups, to families with children who are visually impaired. LOOK also helps to secure appropriate provision for health, welfare, and education

It is important to emphasise to the patient that being registered as blind does not mean that they are totally blind in the lay sense of the word

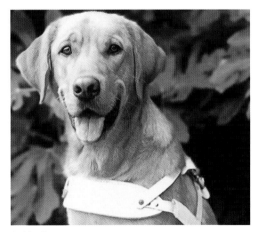
Guide dog

the Guide Dogs for the Blind Association and local voluntary organisations for the visually impaired.

## Visual function and driving

In the United Kingdom the visual standards for driving are applied by the Driver and Vehicle Licensing Agency (DVLA). Different standards apply for drivers of cars or light vehicles and drivers of large goods and passenger vehicles. The following broad areas of visual function are considered:

- Visual acuity
- Visual field
- Vision under conditions of reduced illumination (night vision)
- Other ophthalmic problems (double vision, blepharospasm).

Patients are required to inform the DVLA if they develop an ophthalmic or neurological disease that may influence their eligibility to drive. The ophthalmologist should advise the patient on this.

> **Further information on visual function and driving is available on the DVLA's website at www.dvla.gov.uk (accessed 28 May 2003)**

## Helpful organisations (continued)

**LOOK London**
Kings Avenue School, 127 Park Hill
London SW4 9PA
Tel: 020 8678 0555 (information line)
Provides same support as above, but for London area only

**Macular Disease Society**
Darwin House, 13A Bridge Street, Andover, Hampshire SP10 1BE
Tel: 0845 241 2041
email: info@maculardisease.org
Website: www.maculardisease.org (accessed 28 Nov 2003)
Information and support for people suffering from, or with an interest in, macular disease. Also funds research

**Micro and Anophthalmic Children's Society (MACS)**
1 Skyrmans Fee, Frinton-on-Sea
Essex CO13 0RN
Tel: 0870 600 6227
email: enquiries@macs.org.uk
Website: www.macs.org.uk (accessed 28 Nov 2003)
Support and information for families of children with these eye conditions

**National Blind Children's Society**
Bradbury House, Market Street
Highbridge, Somerset TA9 3BW
Tel: 01278 764764
email: enquiries@nbcs.org.uk
Website: www.nbcs.org.uk (accessed 28 Nov 2003)
Provides the resources to ensure that educational goals can be achieved. Provides grants, advocacy, IT training, and a customised large print book service. Assists children and adults up to age 25

**Nystagmus Network**
13 Tinsley Close, Claypole, Newark, Nottinghamshire NG23 5BS
Tel: 01636 627004
Insight helpline: 01392 272573
email: info@nystagmusnet.org
Website: www.nystagmusnet.org (accessed 28 Nov 2003)
Support group for those with the eye condition nystagmus

**Partially Sighted Society**
Queen's Road, Doncaster, South Yorkshire DN1 2NX
Tel: 01302 323132
email: info@partsight.org.uk
Provision of equipment and advice on living and working with impaired vision. Contact main office in Doncaster for local self help branches

**Retinoblastoma Society**
The Royal London Hospital, Whitechapel Road, London E1 1BB
London EC1A 7BE
Tel: 020 7377 5578
email: rbinfo@rbsociety.org.uk
Website: www.rbsociety.org.uk (accessed 28 Nov 2003)
Support and information about this eye cancer for families, carers, and the professionals who work with them

**RLSB (Royal London Society for the Blind)**
Head Office: Dorton House School, Seal
Nr Sevenoaks, Kent TN15 0ED
Tel: 01732 592500
email: dortonhouseschool@compuserve.com
Website: www.rlsb.org.uk (accessed 28 Nov 2003)
RLSB provides a comprehensive service for children and adults with visual impairment. This includes family support, education, further educational support for work placements, and industrial workshops

**RNIB (Royal National Institute for the Blind)**
105 Judd Street, London WC1H 9NE
Helpline: 0845 7669999
Tel: 020 7388 1266
email: helpline@rnib.org.uk
Website: www.rnib.org.uk (accessed 28 Nov 2003)
Provides over 60 services and support for blind and partially sighted people of all ages and their families. RNIB's customer services (tel: 0845 702 3153) can provide a free copy of the publication *Your guide to RNIB services*

**Sense (formerly the National Deafblind and Rubella Association)**
11-13 Clifton Terrace, Finsbury Park London N4 3SR
Tel: 020 7272 7774
email: enquiries@sense.org.uk
Website: www.sense.org.uk (accessed 28 Nov 2003)
Provides services and support to people with multisensory disabilities and their families

**Tadpoles Parent Support Group (International Glaucoma Association)**
108C Warner Road, London SE5 9HQ
Tel: 020 7737 3265
email: info@iga.org.uk
Website: www.iga.org.uk (accessed 28 May 2003)
Support and information for families and carers of children with glaucoma

## Useful publications, media, and services

### Guidelines for health professionals

Summary guidelines for good practice for health professionals involved with newly diagnosed blind or partially sighted children and their families are available:

- Summary guidelines (leaflet)—*Taking the time: telling parents their child is blind or partially sighted* can be obtained free from:
  RNIB Children's Policy Unit, 105 Judd Street
  London WCIH 9NE
  Tel: 0207 388 1266
  Website: www.rnib.org.uk
- More detailed guidelines (book)—*Taking the time: telling parents their child is blind or partially sighted* compiled with parents and representatives of more than 20 professional organisations is available from:
  RNIB Customer Services, PO Box 173, Peterborough PE2 6WS
  Tel: 0845 702 3153
  Email: cservices@rnib.org.uk
  Website: www.rnib.org.uk
  Price £10.00; please quote code PR11005

### Talking newspapers and talking books

There is a wide variety of taped services available nationally and locally, some examples of which are given below. All are dispatched under the "Articles for the blind" freepost service

### Calibre

New Road, Weston Turville
Aylesbury, Bucks HP22 5XQ
Tel: 01296 432339
email: name@calibre.org.uk
Website: www.calibre.org.uk (accessed 28 Nov 2003)
Cassette library for visually impaired children and adults

### Clearvision

Linden Lodge School, 61 Princes Way
London SW19 6JB
Tel: 020 8789 9575
Nationwide lending library of braille and print children's books

### Talking Newspapers Association of the UK (TNAUK)

National Recording Centre, Heathfield
East Sussex TN21 8DB
Tel: 01435 866102
email: info@tnauk.org.uk
Website: www.tnauk.org.uk (accessed 28 Nov 2003)
Supplies subscription service for over 200 titles nationally and provides local service, usually free, of 1100 titles. Mainly audio cassettes

### RNIB Talking Books

PO Box 173, Peterborough PE2 6WS
Tel: 0845 762 6843
email: cservices@rnib.org.uk
Website: www.rnib.org.uk
Taped book service requiring special machine with easy to operate controls. Also digital (CD) service

### RNIB Cassette Library

PO Box 173, Peterborough PE2 6WS
Tel: 0845 702 3153
email: cservices@rnib.org.uk
Website: www.rnib.org.uk
Wide range of titles, mainly academic subjects, recorded on standard audio cassettes

### Languages other than English

A growing number of titles are now available in other languages such as Welsh, Gaelic, Hindi, Urdu, Gujerati, and Bengali. Details of these and other tape services can be obtained from RNIB Customer Services: 0845 702 3153
email: cservices@rnib.org.uk
Website: www.rnib.org.uk

### Large print books

These can be borrowed from most public libraries and the RNIB. For a list of books to buy, including titles for children and for visually impaired parents wishing to teach their sighted child, please contact RNIB Customer Services
Tel: 0845 702 3153
email: cservices@rnib.org.uk
Website: www.rnib.org.uk

Books can also be purchased from:

### BBC Audio Books

Windsor Bridge Road, Bath BA2 3AX
Tel: 01225 335336
email: sales@bbc.co.uk
Website: www.chivers.co.uk (accessed 28 Nov 2003)
Provides large-print and talking books

### ISIS Large-print and Audio Books

7 Centremead, Osneymead
Oxford OX2 0ES
Tel: 01865 790358
email: sales@ulverscroft.co.uk
Website: www.ulverscroft.co.uk (accessed 28 Nov 2003)
Publishers of large print books

### Magna

Magna House, Long Preston
Nr Skipton, North Yorkshire BD23 4ND
Tel: 01729 840225
email: dallen@magnaprint.co.uk
Website: www.ulverscroft.co.uk (accessed 28 May 2003)
Provides wide range of fiction in large-print books, tapes, and CDs

### Ulverscroft Large-print Books Ltd

The Green, Bradgate Road, Anstey
Leicester LE7 7FU
Tel: 0116 236 4325
email: enquiries@ulverscroft.co.uk
Website: www.ulverscroft.co.uk (accessed 28 Nov 2003)

### Radio programme

*In touch*
This radio programme is broadcast weekly on BBC Radio 4 and reports on issues that affect the lives of visually impaired people in the United Kingdom.

### Specialist centres

In most towns there are specialist centres where blind and partially sighted people can obtain information, examine, and sometimes buy equipment suited to their needs. The facilities that centres provide vary widely. They are mainly run by local voluntary societies for the visually impaired

# 8 Cataracts

"Cataract" describes any lens opacity—from the smallest dot to complete opacification. The prevalence of cataracts increases with age: 65% of people aged 50 to 59 have opacities, and all people aged over 80. An operation is only considered when the opacities substantially interfere with vision. Cataracts are the major cause of blindness in the world today.

## Symptoms

Symptoms depend on whether the cataracts are unilateral or bilateral and the degree and position of the opacity. If the cataract is unilateral the patient may not notice its effects until they have cause to cover the good eye. Patients may complain of difficulty in reading (which should be differentiated from presbyopia that is normal in older people), in recognising faces (which also occurs in macular degeneration), and in watching television. They may complain that their vision worsens in bright light, especially if their opacity is central.

Occasionally patients experience monocular diplopia and see haloes around lights; this occurs because the lens opacity interferes with light rays passing to the back of the eye. Some patients may even report that they can read without glasses. This happens when a nuclear sclerotic cataract increases the converging power of the lens, so making the patient myopic (shortsighted).

## Signs

Although cataracts are common, they are not the only cause of visual problems. The patient with a cataract should be able to point to the position of a light. Lack of normal "projection of light" may indicate problems either in the posterior part of the eye or beyond. The pupillary reactions should also be normal. If they are not, retinal disease or an abnormality of the visual pathway should be suspected.

Cataracts in children are much more serious, as the development of the vision may be impaired irreversibly (visual deprivation amblyopia), even if the cataracts are removed later. Any child with suspected cataracts should be referred immediately. Cataracts in young children are detected by looking at the red reflex (see below), and this should be a routine part of the examination of a young child.

There are three signs of cataract.

### A reduction in visual acuity
The degree of visual impairment depends on the nature of the cataract and the conditions of testing. Visual acuity should also be tested with a pinhole to eliminate the effect of refractive errors.

### A diminished red reflex on ophthalmoscopy
When the ophthalmoscope is used to view the eye from about two feet away, the reflection of the fundus can be seen as a "red reflex." This is the troublesome reflex so often seen in photographs of people taken with a flashlight. If there is any opacity between the cornea and the retina, this reflex will have opacities in it. The nature of the opacities in the reflex will depend on the position and extent of the opacities in the optical media. This reflex is more easily seen when the pupil is dilated.

**Cataracts may cause difficulty in:**

- Reading
- Recognising faces
- Watching television
- Seeing in bright light
- Driving

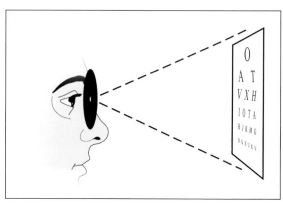

A pinhole improves the visual acuity if the problem is caused by refractive error

**Children with cataracts must be referred immediately**

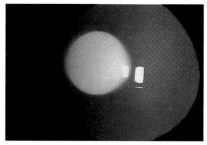

Clear red reflex

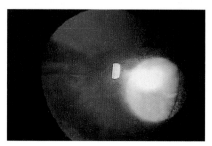

Opacities obscuring red reflex

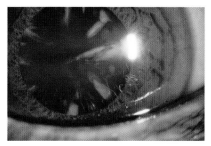

Cortical lens opacity

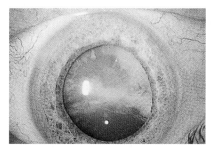

Cortical cataract

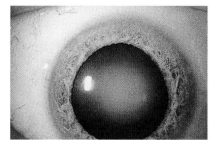

Nuclear sclerotic cataract

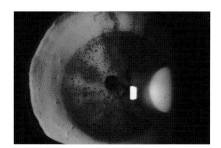

Congenital cataract

*A change in the appearance of the lens*
If you shine a bright light on the eye the lens may appear brown, or even white if the cataract is more advanced.

## Causes

Many conditions are associated with cataracts, but changes within the lens associated with ageing are the most common cause. Cataracts also occur more often in patients with diabetes, uveitis, or a history of trauma to the eye. Prolonged courses of steroids, both oral and topical, can also give rise to cataracts. Children with cataracts need to be investigated to exclude treatable metabolic conditions such as galactosaemia.

## Surgery

There is no effective medical treatment for established cataracts. The treatment is surgical.

**Indications for cataract surgery**
Whether or not to operate depends primarily on the effect of the cataracts on the patient's vision. Many years ago surgeons waited until the cataract was mature or "ripe" (when the contents became liquefied) because this made aspiration of the contents of the lens easier. With advances in microsurgery, however, there is now no longer any need to wait for the cataract to mature, and cataract surgery can be performed at any stage, with minimal risk.

There is no set level of vision for which an operation is essential, but most patients with a vision of 6/18 or worse in both eyes because of lens opacities benefit from cataract extraction. Some elderly patients, however, may be perfectly happy with this level of vision. Simple advice such as the recommendation to use a good reading light that provides illumination from above and behind, may be adequate.

A younger patient, with more exacting visual demands, may opt for an operation much earlier. (The minimum standard for driving is about 6/10; equivalent to a line between 6/9 and 6/12.) With certain types of cataract, such as an opacity at the

**Causes of acquired cataract include:**
- Age
- Diabetes
- Inflammation
- Trauma
- Steroids

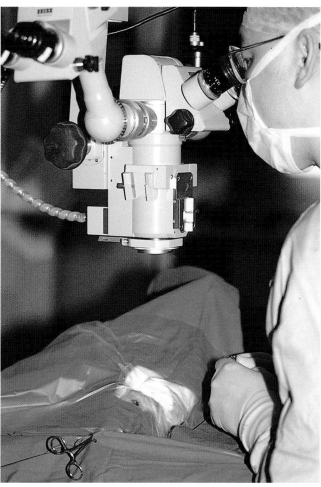

Binocular operating microscope in position at the start of surgery

back of the lens (posterior subcapsular cataract) the vision may be 6/6 in dim conditions when the pupil is dilated. However, in bright sunlight the pupil constricts and most of the light entering the eye has to pass through the opacity, causing glare and a fall in acuity. In this case, surgery would usually be performed even though the tested vision was 6/6. Generally, the surgeon's advice is tailored to the individual patient.

### Surgical techniques
#### "Phacoemulsification" method
Most cataract surgery in the United Kingdom is now performed with this method. A very small tunnel incision (about 3 mm wide) is made in the eye and a circular hole (diameter about 5 mm) is made in the anterior capsule of the lens (capsulorrhexis). A fine ultrasonic probe is then used to liquefy the hard lens nucleus (phacoemulsification) through this hole. Any remaining soft lens fibres then are aspirated. A folded replacement lens is then inserted into the empty lens capsular bag and allowed to unfold. A high viscosity gel substance (viscoelastic) often is used to protect the delicate endothelial cells that line the posterior surface of the cornea during the operation. This is then washed out at the end of the procedure. Sutures often are not required as the tunnel incision is self sealing. These advances in technique have considerably improved the speed of recovery and visual rehabilitation after cataract surgery.

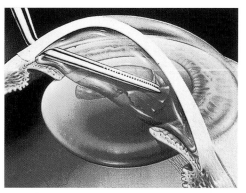

Removal of the anterior capsule of the lens (capsulorrhexis)

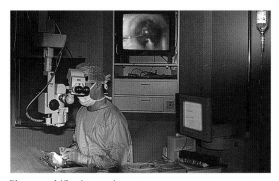

Phacoemulsification equipment

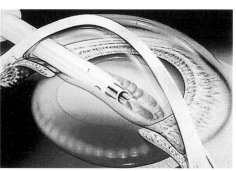

Liquefaction of lens nucleus with an ultrasonic probe through a 2-3 mm incision (phacoemulsification)

#### Extracapsular method
This was, until recently, the most popular method of cataract extraction. An incision is made in the eye (about 10 mm in length) and the anterior capsule is cut open with the tip of a sharp needle. The large nucleus is then expressed whole and the remaining soft lens fibres aspirated. A non-folding lens is then inserted into the empty lens capsular bag and the incision closed with fine sutures. The need for a larger wound in extracapsular surgery may lead to problems with wound security and postoperative astigmatism in some patients.

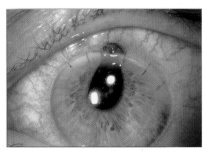

Extracapsular iris prolapse

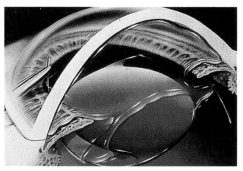

Plastic lens being inserted into the remaining clear capsular bag of the natural lens

*Intracapsular method*

In this method, the entire lens is removed within its capsule, usually with a cryoprobe, after the suspensory ligaments of the lens have been dissolved by the enzyme chymotrypsin. As there is no remaining lens capsule, the vitreous gel in the eye can move forward and block the flow of aqueous through the pupil. A hole cut in the iris (iridectomy) allows the aqueous to bypass the pupil. This method is now usually used only in special situations.

## Anaesthesia

For most patients, cataract surgery is carried out under local anaesthesia as a day case. Local anaesthetic can be injected around the eye (peribulbar anaesthesia or sub-Tenon's anaesthesia), or, with modern, closed system, small incision, cataract surgery, the operation can be carried out safely in selected patients with just topical (eyedrop) anaesthesia. Occasionally, intraocular (intracameral) local anaesthesia is used. In certain situations general anaesthesia may be needed because of anticipated technical difficulties or because of patient factors (for example, in patients with Down's syndrome or young patients who are not cooperative).

## Intraocular lens implants

The final refractive state of the eye after operation can be chosen by measuring the curvature of the cornea (keratometry) and the length of the eye (ultrasound biometry) and then implanting a lens of appropriate power. An intraocular lens implant can be more effective in correcting refractive error than glasses and contact lenses, as it is placed in the eye in the same position as the natural lens.

Myopia and hypermetropia can be corrected during cataract surgery by inserting an appropriately powered intraocular lens. However, patients usually still require glasses for reading or distance, as most implanted lenses have a fixed focus. Multifocal intraocular lenses have two principal points of focus and in theory enable the patient to have both good distance and reading vision without glasses. However, some patients experience optical aberrations and a reduction in contrast sensitivity with this type of intraocular lens.

Most lenses implanted nowadays are posterior chamber lenses, which are placed in the empty lens capsular bag after the lens contents have been removed from the eye. With this type of lens the lens implant sits in a natural position. These lenses can be folded and inserted through a minute incision (2-3 mm). If the lens capsule is not present or cannot support a posterior chamber lens unaided, the lens can be sutured in place. Alternatively, an anterior chamber lens, which is supported in the anterior chamber angle, can be used. In the past, iris clip lenses were used, but they are not used now. The pupil should not be dilated if the iris clip type of lens has been used, as the lens may dislocate.

> Cataract surgery with lens implantations can be combined with other intraocular surgery if necessary, including glaucoma drainage or corneal graft surgery

# Complications of cataract surgery

Over 200 000 cataract operations are performed annually in the United Kingdom, and although modern surgical techniques have exceptional levels of safety, complications still occur. Patient expectations of cataract surgery are very high. All patients should be made aware of the possible risks of the surgery before they give their consent for the operation.

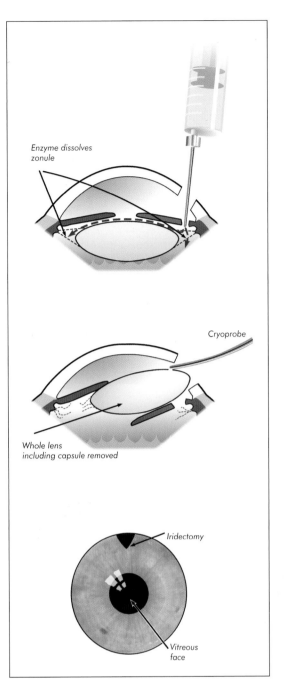

Enzyme dissolves zonule

Cryoprobe

Whole lens including capsule removed

Iridectomy

Vitreous face

Intracapsular cataract surgery

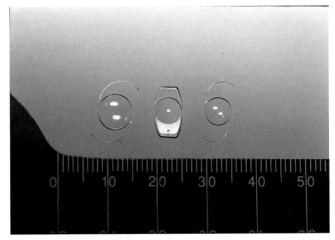

Left: large perspex lens for extracapsular surgery. Middle: silicone foldable lens. Right: small perspex lens, both for photoemulsification

### Infective endophthalmitis

This devastating infection occurs very rarely (about 1 in 1000 operations) but can cause permanent severe reduction of vision. Most cases of postoperative infection present within two weeks of surgery. Typically patients present with a short history of a reduction in their vision and a red painful eye. This is an ophthalmic emergency. Low grade infection with pathogens such as *Propionibacterium* species can lead patients to present several weeks after initial surgery with a refractory uveitis.

### Suprachoroidal haemorrhage

Severe intraoperative bleeding can lead to serious and permanent reduction in vision.

### Ocular perforation

Sharp needles are used for many forms of ocular anaesthesia, and globe perforation is a rare possibility. Modern forms of ocular anaesthesia have replaced many sharp needle techniques.

### Retinal detachment

This serious postoperative complication is, fortunately, rare but is more common in myopic (shortsighted) patients after intraoperative complications.

### Postoperative refractive error

Most operations aim to leave the patient emmetropic or slightly myopic, but in rare cases biometric errors can occur or an intraocular lens of incorrect power is used. Despite all efforts to produce accurate biometry, in occasional cases the desired refractive outcome is not achieved.

### Posterior capsular rupture and vitreous loss

If the very delicate capsular bag is damaged during surgery or the fine ligaments (zonule) suspending the lens are weak (for example, in pseudoexfoliation syndrome), then the vitreous gel may prolapse into the anterior chamber. This complication may mean that an intraocular lens cannot be inserted at the time of surgery. Patients are also at increased risk of postoperative retinal detachment.

### Uveitis

Postoperative inflammation is more common in certain types of eyes for example in patients with diabetes or previous ocular inflammatory disease.

### Cystoid macular oedema

Accumulation of fluid at the macula postoperatively can reduce the vision in the first few weeks after successful cataract surgery. In most cases this resolves with treatment of the post-operative inflammation.

### Glaucoma

Persistently elevated intraocular pressure may need treatment postoperatively.

### Posterior capsular opacification

Scarring of the posterior part of the capsular bag, behind the intraocular lens, occurs in up to 20% of patients. Laser capsulotomy may be needed (see Thickening of the lens capsule, below).

## Postoperative care

Most patients are treated for several weeks with steroid drops to reduce inflammation and with antibiotic drops to prevent infection. Patients have traditionally been advised to avoid activities that may considerably raise the pressure in the eyeball, such as strenuous exercise or heavy lifting, for a few weeks after the operation. However, with modern small incision surgery

**Postoperative infective endophthalmitis is an ophthalmic emergency**

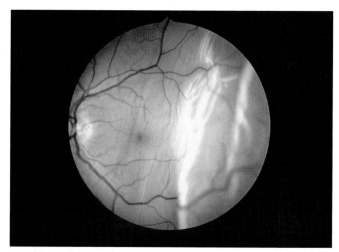

Retinal detachment

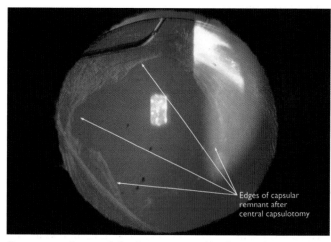

Edges of capsular remnant after central capsulotomy

Opaque posterior capsule has been cut away with a laser to clear the visual axis

**Postoperative care after cataract surgery**

- Steroid drops (inflammation)
- Antibiotic drops (infection)
- Avoid very strenuous exertion and ocular trauma

patients can return to normal activities within a few weeks. If sutures have been necessary, these often need to be taken out before glasses can be prescribed because of the changes they induce in the shape and refractive state of the eye.

*Thickening of the lens capsule*

The remaining lens capsule may thicken (usually over months or years) and this may need to be cut open. In patients who have had previous cataract surgery, capsular thickening is the most common cause of gradually worsening vision. Division of this thickened capsule (capsulotomy) is usually done with a special laser (called the Q-switched neodymium yttrium-aluminium-garnet or Nd-YAG laser), which creates microscopic focused explosions that dissect tissue rather than burn it. This avoids the need to open the eye surgically, and it can be performed painlessly (the capsule has no pain fibres) on an outpatient basis, under topical anaesthesia, with the patient sitting at a slit-lamp microscope. This treatment has given rise in part to patients' commonly held misconception that cataracts can be removed by laser alone.

# Optical correction after surgery

Removal of the crystalline lens results in an eye with a large hypermetropic refractive error. This refractive error is usually corrected with an intraocular lens implant at the time of surgery. If the implant results in clear vision for distance, glasses usually will be required for reading fine print, as the new lens has a fixed focus. If the patient had a cataract extraction before intraocular lenses were used commonly, optical correction has to be achieved with glasses or a contact lens.

*Glasses*

The natural lens has great refractive power and consequently the glasses required to correct the refractive error after cataract extraction are thick and heavy, even when they are made of plastic. The corrected image is about 30% larger than that seen by the normal eye. This means that the image from an eye that has had a cataract removed, with subsequent glasses correction, cannot be fused with the image from the other eye, unless the lens in the other eye is also removed. Objects are also perceived to be closer than they are, often resulting in accidents—for example, pouring tea into the lap rather than into the cup. The field of vision is restricted, and there is a "blind ring" (scotoma) within this field because of the optical aberrations inherent in such powerful lenses. These optical problems do not occur with contact lenses or an intraocular lens implant.

*Contact lenses*

The size of an image with a contact lens is only 10% larger than the image in the normal eye. The brain can fuse this disparity and thus both an operated eye and an unoperated eye may be used simultaneously. However, most patients with cataracts are elderly and problems may arise in using the contact lens because of an inadequate tear film, difficulties with handling, and infection.

*Secondary intraocular lens implantation*

If the problems posed by using glasses or contact lenses are too great, secondary implantation of an intraocular lens can be considered. However, this procedure has associated risks, particularly in patients who have had intracapsular cataract extraction. Complications may occur, including secondary glaucoma. The potential advantages and disadvantages of the various options need to be fully considered by the patient and the ophthalmologist before a final decision is made.

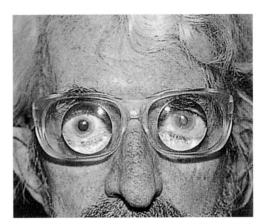

Cataract glasses—thick, heavy, expensive, with magnified image and reduced field of vision—are now rarely necessary because of intraocular lens implants

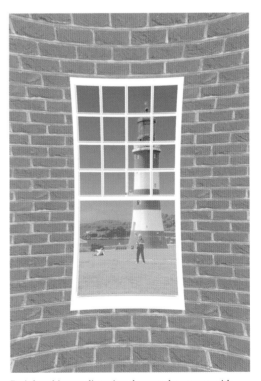

Peripheral image distortion that may be present with cataract glasses

# 9 Glaucoma

The glaucomas are a range of disorders with a characteristic type of optic nerve damage. The glaucomas are the second commonest cause of blindness in the world, and the commonest cause of irreversible blindness. The most effective way of preventing this damage is to lower the intraocular pressure.

Normally the ciliary body secretes aqueous, which flows into the posterior chamber and through the pupil into the anterior chamber. It leaves the eye through the trabecular meshwork, flowing into Schlemm's canal and into episcleral veins. The flow and drainage can be obstructed in several ways.

## Symptoms and signs

A patient with primary open angle glaucoma (also known as chronic open angle glaucoma) may not notice any symptoms until severe visual damage has occurred. This is because the rise in intraocular pressure and consequent damage occurs so slowly that the patient has time to compensate. In contrast, the clinical presentation of acute angle closure glaucoma is well known, as the intraocular pressure rises rapidly and results in a red, painful eye with disturbance of vision.

> **The clinical signs of raised intraocular pressure depend on both the rate and degree of the rise in pressure**

### Raised intraocular pressure

Most patients with raised intraocular pressure (IOP) are unaware that they have a problem. Raised IOP is detected most commonly through screening as part of a routine eye test by an optometrist. The IOP is determined by the balance between aqueous production inside the eye and aqueous drainage out of the eye through the trabecular meshwork. Each normal eye makes about 2 μl of aqueous a minute—that is, about 70 litres during the course of a lifetime. In a British Caucasian population, 95% of people have an IOP between 10 and 21 mm Hg, but IOP can drop as low as 0 mm Hg in hypotony and can exceed 70 mm Hg in some glaucomas.

The rate at which raised IOP causes optic nerve damage depends on many factors, including the level of IOP and whether glaucomatous damage is early or advanced. In general, raised IOPs in the 20-30 mm Hg range usually cause damage over several years, but very high IOPs in the 40-50 mm Hg range can cause rapid visual loss and also precipitate retinovascular occlusion.

### Haloes around lights and a cloudy cornea

The cornea is kept transparent by the continuous removal of fluid by the endothelial cells. If the pressure rises slowly, this process takes longer to fail. When the pressure rises quickly (acute closed angle glaucoma) the cornea becomes waterlogged, causing a fall in visual acuity and creating haloes around lights (like looking at a light through frosted glass).

### Pain

If the rise in pressure is slow, pain is not a feature of glaucoma until the pressure is extremely high. Pain is not characteristically a feature of primary open angle glaucoma.

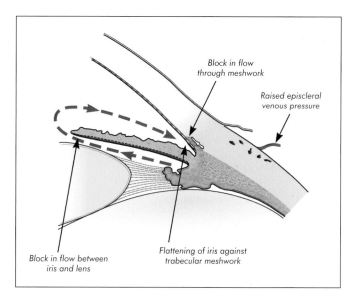

Normal aqueous drainage and possible sites of obstruction

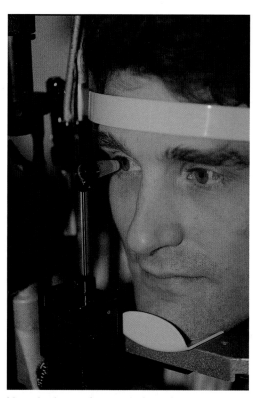

Measuring intraocular pressure by applanation tonometry

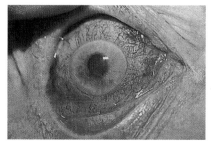

Cloudy cornea after sudden rise in intraocular pressure (acute angle closure glaucoma)

*Visual field loss*

Pressure on the nerve fibres and chronic ischaemia at the optic nerve head cause damage to the retinal nerve fibres and usually results in characteristic patterns of field loss (arcuate scotoma).

However, this spares central vision initially, and the patient does not notice the defect. Sophisticated visual field testing techniques are required to detect early visual field defects. The terminal stage of glaucomatous field loss is a severely contracted field, because only a few fibres from the more richly innervated macula area survive. Even at this stage (tunnel vision) the vision may still be 6/6.

*Optic disc changes*

The optic disc marks the exit point of the retinal nerve fibres from the eye. With a sustained rise in IOP the nerve fibres atrophy, leaving the characteristic sign of chronic glaucoma—the cupped, pale optic disc.

*Venous occlusion*

Raised IOP can impede blood flow in the low pressure venous system, increasing the risk of retinal venous occlusion.

*Enlargement of the eye*

In adults no significant enlargement of the eye is possible because growth has ceased. In a young child there may be enlargement of the eye (buphthalmos or "ox-eye"). This tends to occur with raised IOP in children under the age of three years. These children may also be photophobic and have watering eyes and cloudy corneas.

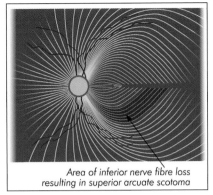

Area of inferior nerve fibre loss resulting in superior arcuate scotoma

Normal distribution of nerve fibres in the retina

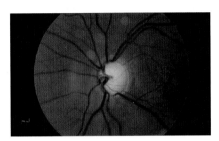

Glaucomatous cupping of the optic nerve

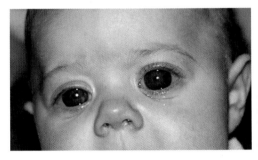

Enlarged watering eyes with cloudy corneas in a child with glaucoma

# Primary open angle glaucoma

Primary open angle glaucoma is the most common form of glaucoma and is the third most common cause of registration of blindness in the United Kingdom. The resistance to outflow through the trabecular meshwork gradually increases, for reasons not fully understood, and the pressure in the eye slowly increases, causing damage to the nerve. The level of IOP is the major risk factor for visual loss. There may be other damage mechanisms, particularly ischaemia of the optic nerve head.

*Symptoms*

Because the visual loss is gradual, patients do not usually present until severe damage has occurred. The disease can be detected by screening high risk groups for the signs of glaucoma. At present most patients with primary open angle glaucoma are detected by optometrists at routine examinations.

*Groups at risk*

The prevalence increases with age from 0.02% in the 40-49 age group to 10% in those aged over 80. Those with an increased

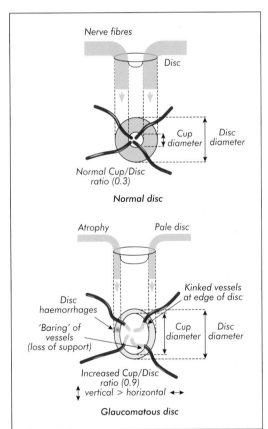

Optic disc changes in glaucoma

**Risk factors for primary open angle glaucoma**

- Level of intraocular pressure
- Increasing age
- African-Caribbean origin
- Family history
- Thin corneas

risk include first degree relatives of patients (1 in 10), patients with ocular hypertension (particularly those with thin corneas, larger cup to disc ratios and higher IOPs), people with myopia, and people of African-Caribbean origin (×5 risk in Caucasians). Recently, genetic mutations have been identified that account for 3-4% of primary open angle glaucomas.

*Signs*

The eye is white and on superficial examination looks normal. The best signs for the purpose of detection are the optic disc changes. The cup to disc ratio increases as the nerve fibres atrophy. Asymmetry of disc cupping is also important, as the disease often is more advanced in one eye than the other. Haemorrhages on the optic disc are a poor prognostic sign. Longer term changes in disc cupping are best detected by serial photography, and the more recently introduced scanning laser ophthalmoscope may be able to detect structural changes in the nerve at an early stage of the disease.

Visual field loss is difficult to pick up clinically without specialised equipment until considerable damage (loss of up to 50% of the nerve fibres) has occurred. Computerised field testing equipment may detect nerve fibre damage earlier, particularly if certain types of stimuli such as fine motion or blue on yellow targets are used. Computer assisted field testing is also the best method for detecting long term change and deterioration of visual fields.

The classical signs of glaucoma (field loss and optic disc cupping) often are seen in patients who have pressures lower than the statistical upper limit of normal (21 mm Hg). However, many clinicians now feel that these two glaucomas are part of the same spectrum of pressure dependent optic neuropathies, although these patients are sometimes referred to as having normal tension glaucoma. For an accurate measurement of IOP, intraocular pressure phasing, taking multiple measurements throughout the day is useful, so that any spikes can be detected.

In normal tension glaucoma there may be a significant component of vascular associated damage at the optic nerve head (ischaemia or vasospasm). Management of progressive normal tension glaucoma involves lowering IOP. Drug induced nocturnal hypotension should be considered in progressive normal tension glaucoma.

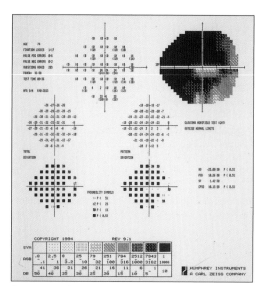

Computerised visual field test print out showing "tunnel" vision

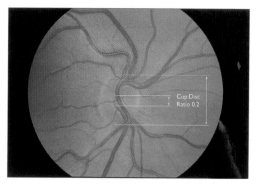

Normal optic disc

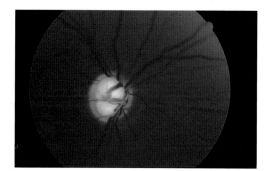

Cupped optic disc

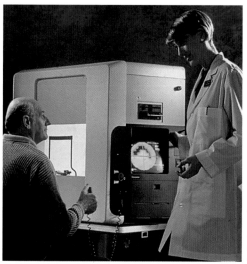

Visual field testing with computerised field testing equipment

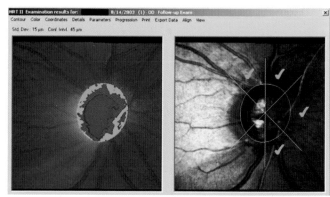

Advanced scanning laser image of cupped optic nerve head

# Acute angle closure glaucoma

Acute angle closure glaucoma is probably the best known type of glaucoma, as the presentation is acute and the affected

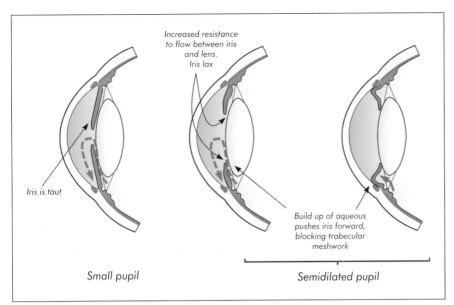

Acute angle closure glaucoma

eye becomes red and painful. In angle closure glaucoma, apposition of the lens to the back of the iris prevents the flow of aqueous from the posterior chamber to the anterior chamber. This is more likely to occur when the pupil is semi dilated at night. Aqueous then collects behind the iris and pushes it on to the trabecular meshwork, preventing the drainage of aqueous from the eye, so the IOP rises rapidly.

*Symptoms*

The eye becomes red and painful because of the rapid rise in IOP, and there is often vomiting. Vision is blurred because the cornea is becoming oedematous; patients may notice haloes around lights due to the dispersion of light through the waterlogged cornea. They may have a history of similar attacks in the past that were aborted by going to sleep. During sleep the pupil constricts and may pull the peripheral iris out of the angle.

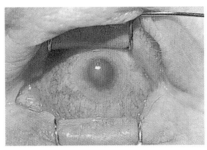

Acute angle closure glaucoma

*Groups at risk*

This type of glaucoma usually occurs in longsighted people (hypermetropes), who tend to have shallow anterior chambers and shorter axial length eyes. With increasing age the lens tends to increase in size and crowd the anterior segment structures in these eyes. Women have shallower anterior chambers and live longer and therefore are more at risk of this type of glaucoma.

For acute angle closure glaucoma, emergency treatment is required to preserve the sight of the eye

*Signs*

Visual acuity is impaired, depending on the degree of corneal oedema. The eye is red and tender to touch. The cornea is hazy because of oedema, and the pupil is semidilated and fixed to light. The attack begins with the pupil in the semidilated position and the rise in pressure makes the iris ischaemic and fixed in that position. On gentle palpation the affected eye feels much harder than the other. Patients often are systemically unwell with nausea, vomiting, and severe pain or headache.

If the patient is seen shortly after an attack has resolved, none of these signs may be present, hence the importance of the history.

*Management*

Emergency treatment is required to preserve the sight of the eye. If it is not possible to get the patient to hospital immediately, acetazolamide 500 mg should be given intravenously, and pilocarpine 4% instilled in the eye to constrict the pupil.

The IOP must first be brought down medically, and a hole (peripheral iridotomy) subsequently must be made in the peripheral iris, either with a laser or surgically, in order to

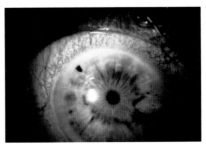

Hole made in the iris (iridotomy) with the Neodymium yttrium-aluminium-garnet (Nd-YAG) laser without having to cut into the eyeball

restore aqueous flow. The other eye should be treated similarly, as a prophylactic measure.

If the treatment is delayed, adhesions may form between the iris and the cornea (peripheral anterior synechiae) and the trabecular meshwork itself may be damaged. A surgical drainage procedure may then be required. Angle closure glaucoma is a very serious condition and even with optimum management the patient may need multiple surgical procedures and have impaired vision. Sometimes laser burns can be made on the iris (iridoplasty) without creating a full thickness hole in the iris. This treatment causes the iris to contract away from the occluded drainage angle.

## Other types of glaucoma

If there is inflammation in the eye (anterior uveitis), adhesions may develop between the lens and iris (posterior synechiae). These adhesions will block the flow of aqueous between the posterior and anterior chambers and result in forward ballooning of the iris and a rise in the IOP. Adhesions may also develop between the iris and cornea (peripheral anterior synechiae), covering up the trabecular drainage meshwork. Inflammatory cells may also block the meshwork. Topical steroids may cause a gradual asymptomatic rise in IOP that can lead to blindness. (Patients taking topical steroids over a long period should always be under ophthalmological supervision.)

The growth of new vessels on the iris (rubeosis) occurs both in diabetic patients and after occlusion of the central retinal vein resulting from retinal ischaemia. These vessels also block the trabecular meshwork causing rubeotic glaucoma, which is extremely difficult to treat.

The trabecular meshwork itself may have developed abnormally (congenital glaucoma) or been damaged by trauma to the eye. Patients who have had eye injuries have a higher chance than normal of developing glaucoma later in life. If there is a bleed in the eye after trauma, the red cells may also block the trabecular meshwork.

## Medical treatment

The main aim of therapy in glaucoma management is reduction of IOP. There is now good evidence from multiple large randomised trials that reducing IOP is effective in preventing disease progression in ocular hypertension, primary open angle glaucoma, and even in so-called normal tension glaucoma. Target pressures in the low teens are associated with the lowest progression rates.

*β blockers (for example, timolol, levobunolol, carteolol, betaxolol, and metipranolol)*
These reduce the secretion of aqueous and are still the most commonly prescribed topical treatment. Contraindications to their use include a history of lung or heart disease, as the drops may cause systemic β blockade. It is important to be aware that topical β blockers can unmask latent and previously undiagnosed chronic obstructive airway disease in elderly people. Systemic effects from eye drops can be reduced by occlusion of the punctum (finger pressed on the caruncle, which can be felt as a lump at the inner canthus of the eye) or shutting the eyes for several minutes after putting in the drops. This reduces the lacrimal pumping mechanism and stops the eyedrops running down the lacrimal passages and being absorbed systemically via the nasal mucosa or by inhalation directly into the lungs. This may also enhance ocular absorption of the drugs. These drops are usually given twice a

---

**Effects of topical steroids**

- Topical steroids may cause a change in the drainage meshwork, resulting in a slow rise in intraocular pressure
- Patients may not complain of visual symptoms until severe damage has occurred

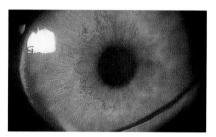

New vessels on the iris causing rubeotic glaucoma

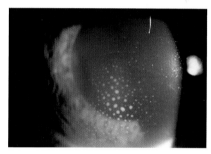

Keratic precipitates

It is important to remember that drops used to treat glaucoma contain powerful drugs that can have marked systemic side effects, despite the low topical doses used

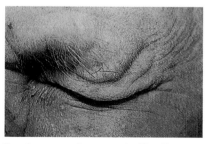

Eye closure to reduce systemic side effects after instilling drops

day, but long acting forms now available can be given once a day, either alone or in combination with other drops.

*Prostaglandin analogues (for example, latanoprost, travoprost, and bimatoprost)*

These reduce the IOP by increasing aqueous outflow from the eye via an alternative drainage route called the uveoscleral pathway. It is possible to get reductions in IOP of up to 30–35% with these drugs. This ability to achieve larger reductions in IOP with improved systemic safety profiles has been a major therapeutic advance in glaucoma. Systemic side effects are minimal but an unusual side effect in a few patients with light irides is a gradual, permanent darkening of the iris. Patients often notice that their eyelashes increase in length and darken. For optimum effect, these drops are used once daily (at night).

*Sympathomimetic agents*

Topical adrenaline, once commonly prescribed, is now rarely used because of lack of efficacy compared with $\beta$ blockers and adverse effects on the conjunctiva. A newer generation of agents that stimulate the $\alpha$ receptors of the sympathetic system is now used—for example, brimonidine (used twice a day) or apraclonidine. Contraindications include cardiovascular disease, because of the potential systemic sympathomimetic effects.

*Parasympathomimetic agents (for example, pilocarpine)*

These constrict the pupil and "pull" on the trabecular meshwork, increasing the flow of the aqueous out of the eye. The small pupil may, however, cause visual problems if central lens opacities are present. Constriction of the ciliary body causes accommodation and blurred vision in young patients. Pilocarpine should not be used if there is inflammation in the eye, as the pupil may stick to the lens close to the visual axis (posterior synechiae) and affect vision. Pilocarpine is usually administered four times a day but can be used twice daily in a combined form with a $\beta$ blocker, or once at night in a gel preparation, which reduces side effects. When patients first instill pilocarpine they often experience a marked brow ache, which tends to reduce with longer term use of the drug. Pilocarpine therapy can increase the risk of retinal detachment.

*Carbonic anhydrase inhibitors*

These are available as topical (for example, dorzolamide, brinzolamide) or oral (for example, acetazolamide) agents. They reduce the secretion of aqueous, and the systemic form, administered orally, is the most powerful agent for reducing IOP, although unfortunately it may have side effects, including nausea, lassitude, paraesthesiae, electrolyte disturbances, and renal stones. The topical form has minimal systemic side effects. Carbonic anhydrase inhibitors should not be used in patients with sulphonamide allergy.

*Neuroprotective agents*

Experimental evidence exists that some neuroprotective agents may reduce intraocular pressure induced glaucomatous damage. However, at present there is no conclusive evidence that these agents are helpful in glaucoma, but large scale clinical trials are currently being carried out in this area.

## Allergy to glaucoma drops

The main symptoms of drop allergy are intense itching and irritation of the eyes and eyelids, which are exacerbated by instillation of the drops. The characteristic signs of drop hypersensitivity include red injected eyes, red swollen eyelids, and ezcema like excoriation of the eyelids and periocular skin.

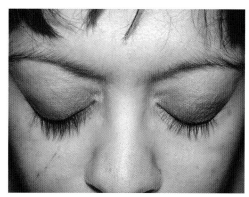

Longer, thicker lashes on right eyelid after prostaglandin treatment

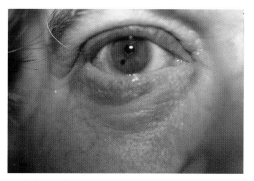

Small pupil with pilocarpine drops

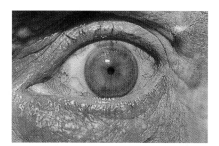

Mild allergy to the active drug component of a glaucoma medication

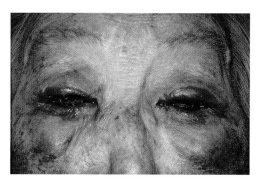

Severe allergy: bilateral allergic dermatitis secondary to the preservation component in a glaucoma drop

The patient may be hypersensitive to the active glaucoma drug or one of the preservative agents used to stabilise the preparation (usually benzalkonium chloride).

The diagnostic test for drop hypersensitivity is controlled cessation of therapy. Symptoms and signs should rapidly improve on withdrawal of the topical therapy. When patients are on multiple topical agents it can be difficult to isolate the agent responsible for the allergic reaction. In cases of allergy to the preservative agent in the drugs, some topical drugs used in glaucoma management are available in preservative free form.

## Laser treatment

### Laser trabeculoplasty

Argon or diode laser "burns" are applied to the trabecular meshwork. How this treatment works is uncertain. It was thought to contract one part of the meshwork, so stretching and opening up adjacent areas, but a more recent hypothesis is that it rejuvenates the cells in the trabecular meshwork. This treatment is used only in the types of glaucoma where the drainage angle is open. Its effect is relatively short term, so this treatment is mainly used for more elderly patients.

### Laser iridotomy

Peripheral laser iridotomy (PI) can be performed in cases of angle closure glaucoma with the Nd-YAG laser, which (unlike argon or diode lasers) actually cuts holes in tissue rather than just burning. This procedure can be performed without incising the eye.

### Laser iridoplasty

Argon laser iridoplasty is a useful procedure in some forms of angle closure glaucoma. A ring of laser burns is applied to the peripheral iris, causing contraction of tissue. This pulls the peripheral iris away from the drainage angle and helps to reduce angle occlusion.

### Laser ciliary body ablation

Lasers can be used to burn the circular ciliary body that produces the aqueous humour. At the correct wavelength the laser radiation passes through the white sclera and is only absorbed by the pigmented ciliary body (transcleral ciliary body cycloablation). This treatment is now commonly performed with a diode laser and usually has to be repeated to maintain lowering of IOP. Most patients undergoing laser ciliary body ablation need to continue medical therapy. Laser destruction of the ciliary body usually is used only in advanced refractory glaucomas or where other surgical options are limited.

## Surgical treatment

Surgery was traditionally used only when treatment had failed to halt the progress of glaucoma, but there is some evidence that earlier surgical intervention is beneficial for selected patients.

### Iridectomy

Peripheral iridectomy is performed in cases of angle closure glaucoma, both in the affected eye and prophylactically in the other eye. Most of these cases can be treated with the Nd-YAG laser. Surgery is reserved for difficult or refractory cases.

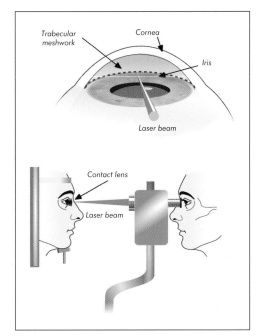

Laser trabeculoplasty

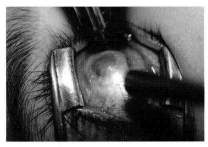

Diode laser with transillumination to locate ciliary body

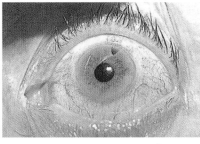

Surgical peripheral iridotomy

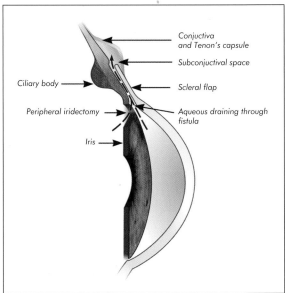

Trabeculectomy

*Drainage surgery*

When it is not possible to achieve the target IOP with medical (or laser) therapy in glaucoma, then the next line of management is surgical. The most effective glaucoma filtration procedure is trabeculectomy. In this procedure a guarded channel is created, which allows aqueous to flow from the anterior chamber inside the eye into the sub-Tenon's and subconjunctival space (bypassing the blocked trabecular meshwork). A drainage "bleb" (aqueous under the conjunctiva and Tenon's capsule) can often be seen under the upper lid. Conjunctivitis in a patient with a drainage bleb should always be treated promptly, as there is an increased risk of the infection entering the eye (endophthalmitis).

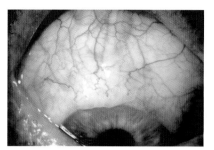

Bleb

## Possible complications

The main cause of surgical failure is postoperative scarring of the drainage channel and drainage bleb. Scarring can be reduced by using adjuvant antiscarring therapy. Various antiscarring agents are used, including drugs used in anticancer therapy. These are delivered by short applications during surgery to the drainage bed on a sponge or by postoperative injections. The most commonly used drugs are 5-fluorouracil and mitomycin-c.

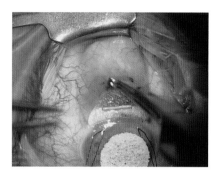

Sponges soaked in 5-fluorourcil to prevent postoperative scarring

Glaucoma filtration procedures do carry some risk and the patient should be advised of the risk of postoperative cataract and hypotony (low pressure) and the possibility of a reduction in postoperative best corrected visual acuity.

Although trabeculectomy remains the gold standard glaucoma filtration procedure, several alternative filtration operations also exist. Non-penetrating deep sclerectomy and viscocanalostomy have good safety profiles but have tended to produce less dramatic reductions in IOP in all published trials.

For certain patients with refractory glaucoma, a tube drainage device may be considered. A drainage tube is inserted, connecting the anterior chamber of the eye with a reservoir in the posterior orbit. This has a good chance of controlling IOP, but also has moderately high risk of serious complications.

## Support group

The International Glaucoma Association is the major support group for patients with glaucoma in the United Kingdom. This organisation provides information pamphlets and support for people with different forms of glaucoma

**International Glaucoma Association**
King's College Hospital
Denmark Hill, London SE5 9RS
Tel/fax: 020 7737 3265
Email: iga@kcl.ac.uk

# 10   Age-related macular degeneration

Age-related macular degeneration (ARMD) is the late stage of age-related maculopathy and the most common cause of blindness in developed countries. The condition is characterised by progressive, bilateral atrophic changes in the choriocapillaris, Bruch's membrane, and the retinal pigment epithelium. The incidence of blinding ARMD increases sharply with increasing age, and it is present in about 15% of all people over the age of 85.

ARMD can be divided clinically into dry (atrophic) and wet (exudative) forms.

### Dry (atrophic, non-exudative) ARMD
This is the common form of ARMD; about 85% of all ARMD is of this type. It is characterised by widespread atrophic changes in the macular area and is bilateral. Dry ARMD usually progresses only slowly and with great variability and may result in severe visual impairment over five to ten years in some patients.

### Wet (exudative, neovascular) ARMD
Wet ARMD is a more aggressive disease and although only 15% of all ARMD cases are of this type, the exudative form is responsible for 90% of all severe visual loss in ARMD. The clinical course of the disease is much more rapid than dry ARMD and 75% of patients will have a marked reduction in vision over about three years. **The chance of second eye involvement in wet ARMD is very high**.

In wet ARMD the problem stems from an abnormal growth of new blood vessels (choroidal neovascularisation) that invade the retina from the choroid. These abnormal blood vessels leak fluid and are associated with bleeding in the macular region.

## Risk factors for ARMD

The aetiology of ARMD is multifactorial and currently is not fully understood. The main risk factor for the development of this degenerative condition seems to be increasing age.

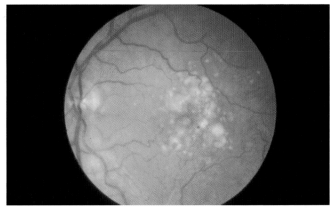

Dry age-related macular degeneration with drusen in the macula area

---

**Various associated risk factors for the development and progression of ARMD have been suggested, including:**

- female sex
- positive smoking history
- positive family history
- hypertension
- raised cholesterol
- history of previous high exposure to ultraviolet light
- hypermetropia
- cataract surgery

---

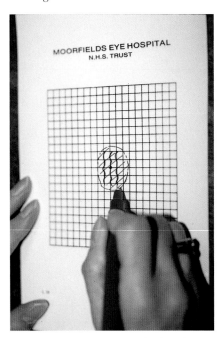

Amsler chart to assess patients who have distortion of their central vision

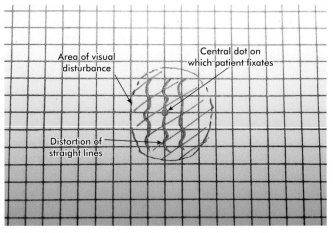

Amsler grid: distortion seen by patient with age-related macular degeneration

# Clinical presentation

Most patients with dry, atrophic ARMD present with a gradual reduction in the **central vision** of both eyes, which affects their ability to read, to recognise faces, and to see clearly in the distance. Patients may notice mild distortion of their central vision (metamorphopsia) but characteristically retain a good peripheral visual field.

In the wet, exudative form of ARMD, patients present more acutely with a sudden change in their central vision (usually in one eye initially). They often experience marked central distortion ("straight lines have a bend in the middle") or a precipitous fall in their vision.

### Signs in dry ARMD

The earliest clinically detectable sign of dry ARMD is the appearance of **drusen** in the macular region of both eyes. Drusen are tiny pinpoint, discrete yellow deposits, which correspond histopathologically to focal accumulations of abnormal hyaline material located specifically at the interface of Bruch's membrane and the retinal pigment epithelium (RPE). Later atrophic changes occur in the macular area, causing a diffuse pale, mottled appearance. This appearance corresponds histopathologically to atrophy of the RPE and choroid, with some areas of secondary RPE hyperplasia. In advanced geographical atrophy of the macula there is a large, well demarcated area of atrophy and it is possible to see clearly the underlying choroidal vessels.

### Signs in wet ARMD

As in dry ARMD, there are drusen and atrophic changes at the macula, but the distinctive signs of wet ARMD relate to the abnormal growth of new blood vessels and leakage of serous fluid and blood into the macula region. Choroidal neovascularisation appears as a small, focal, pale pink-yellow or grey-green elevation at the macula. There may be associated exudation of serous fluid or blood in the subretinal or sub-RPE space.

# Investigation

Fundus fluorescein angiography (FFA), sometimes augmented with indocyanine green angiography (ICG), is used to confirm the presence of an area of choroidal neovascularisation at the macula. In both techniques, intravenous administration of a dye allows assessment of the retinal and choroidal circulations and highlights areas of macular pathology (particularly the presence of abnormal, leaking blood vessels). Fundus fluorescein angiography is a safe and commonly performed investigation in ophthalmic practice. However, very rarely a patient may experience a serious episode of laryngeal oedema, bronchospasm, or anaphylactic shock as a result of the fluorescein injection. On the basis of fluorescein angiography, choroidal neovascularisation can be divided into **classic** (neovascularisation fully delineated) and **occult** (full extent of neovascularisation not visible). The classic form usually progresses faster than the occult form.

# Management of ARMD

The ophthalmologist has a very important role in managing patients with ARMD, even though very little can be done at present to influence the natural progression of the disease in the majority of patients. When told that they have ARMD, most patients will immediately worry about the risk of total

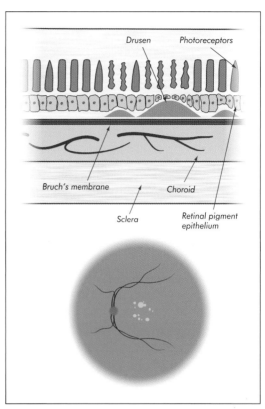

Dry macular degeneration

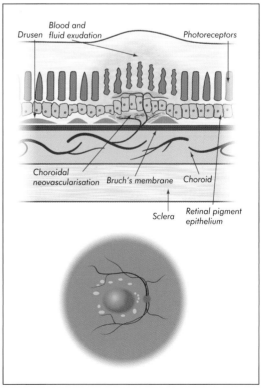

Wet macular degeneration

blindness. Although ARMD will almost certainly cause a progressive reduction in central visual acuity in many patients, the rate of deterioration is extremely variable, and most patients will continue to lead active independent lives with full preservation of their peripheral visual fields. The ophthalmologist has a key role here in demonstrating to the patient that the peripheral visual fields (to confrontation) are full. Together with appropriate information about ARMD and self help groups, this reassurance is the essential component of the consultation.

The patient can be offered visual rehabilitation (refraction and low vision assessment) and registration as partially sighted or blind (see Chapter 7). Specific advice about diet and lifestyle measures can be offered, based on recent research findings in this field. Much interest in recent years has focussed on the possible role of dietary supplementation in ARMD, and recent evidence suggests that the progression of ARMD in some patients can be reduced by vitamin supplementation. A balanced diet (rich in fresh fruit and green leafy vegetables) is important and this can be supplemented by preparations containing multivitamins, vitamin C, vitamin A and beta-carotene, zinc, omega 3 fatty acids (found in fish), lutein, and xeaxanthin.

### Specific management of wet ARMD

Treatments specifically for wet ARMD aim to close off blood flow through the area of choroidal neovascularisation, to allow resolution of the exudative changes at the macula and the restoration of central visual function. The first stage is to determine whether the patient is in the subgroup of ARMD patients for whom ablation of the choroidal neovascularisation is effective. Patients with severe secondary fibrotic changes in the delicate tissues of the macula are less likely to regain visual function through this treatment. The pattern of choroidal neovascularisation, determined using fundus fluorescein angiography and indocyanine green angiography, is also very important. Monitoring of patients who have been treated for wet ARMD is essential, because the choroidal neovascularisation can recur.

Several different methods of ablation of choroidal neovascularisation are available for treating wet ARMD.

#### Laser photocoagulation

The neovascularisation is occluded by direct laser photocoagulation. In the process of destroying the deeper abnormal vessel leakage, the overlying retina also sustains significant damage. This type of treatment is often used for extrafoveal and juxtafoveal choroidal neovascularisation that does not lie directly beneath the fovea. In subfoveal disease laser photocoagulation will result in an immediate reduction in vision.

#### Photodynamic therapy (PDT)

This new technique uses a light activated photosensitiser (verteporfin), given intravenously. An ophthalmic laser delivery system is used to generate the specific wavelength of light to activate the photosensitiser, which causes photochemical damage and vessel occlusion in the selected target area. This makes it possible to cause vessel occlusion without damage to the retina, which has the advantage of preserving visual function, particularly with choroidal neovascularisation in the subfoveal region. PDT has become the treatment of choice in subfoveal choroidal neovascularisation.

**On the basis of FFA findings subfoveal choroidal neovascularisation can be divided into four categories**

- *Classic with no occult*—lesions that are composed of classic choroidal neovascularisation with no evidence of an occult component
- *Predominantly classic with occult*—lesions in which 50% or more of the entire area is classic choroidal neovascularisation but some occult choroidal neovascularisation is present
- *Minimally classic*—lesions in which less that 50% but more than 0% of the area is classic choroidal neovascularisation
- *Occult only*—lesions in which there is occult choroidal neovascularisation with no evidence of classic choroidal neovascularisation

At present the main treatment effect of PDT is seen in classic lesions with no occult

From *Guidance on the use of photodynamic therapy for age-related macular degeneration*. London: NICE, 2003

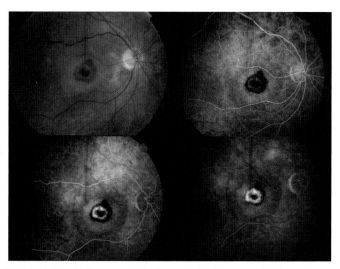

Subfoveal choroidal neovascularisation—classic with no occult. Increasing "lacy" hyperfluorescent dye leakage from the abnormal blood vessels is clearly demarcated

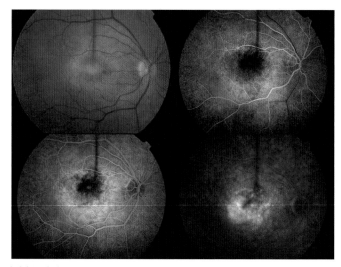

Subfoveal choroidal neovascularisation—occult. Increasing diffuse hyperfluorescent dye leakage with the source of leakage unable to be clearly defined

*External beam radiation*
Precisely focused radiotherapy is used to ablate the neovascular membrane. This treatment is currently undergoing evaluation in certain centres.

*Agents that inhibit choroidal neovascularisation*
A variety of agents that may inhibit subfoveal choroidal neovascularisation are being investigated. These include novel molecules such as antibodies and aptamers (RNA-like molecules). The molecules neutralise growth factors such as vascular endothelial growth factor, which stimulates new vessel growth. Anti-angiogenic steroids are also being tested.

*Submacular surgery*
This is an operation involving microsurgical vitrectomy to remove the vitreous gel, combined with a retinal incision and then removal of the choroidal neovascularisation. This technique may be appropriate for selected cases.

*Macular rotation or transposition surgery*
This is a complex surgical technique in which the macular region of the retina is physically moved to overlie another area of healthy retinal pigment epithelium elsewhere in the adjacent retina. Subsequent strabismus surgery is need to rotate the macula back into the primary position. This complicated operation is still under development and carries significant risk at present.

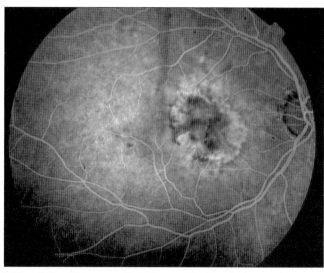

Subfoveal choroidal neovascularisation—predominantly classic with occult

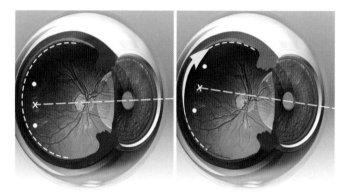

Retinal transposition with macular rotation

# 11   Squint

Many practitioners approach the subject of squint (strabismus) with great trepidation, sometimes with justification. However, if it is approached systematically, much of the myth and mystery can be dispelled.

## What is a squint?

The word is used in many different ways. It is often used to describe the narrowing of the gap between the upper and lower eyelids (interpalpebral fissure), usually carried out by patients to create a pinhole effect. This reduces the consequences of any refractive error, and improves the clarity of the image. However, the true definition of squint is that one of the eyes is not directed towards the object under scrutiny. Note that if the eyes converge for close work, this does not indicate a squint.

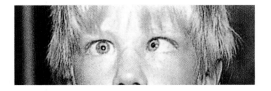

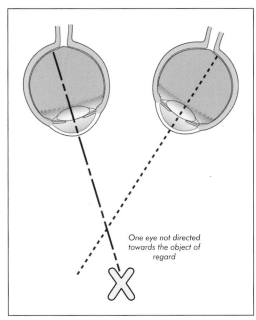

*One eye not directed towards the object of regard*

The true definition of squint

## Why is a squint important?

**A squint may show that the acuity of the eye is impaired** because of ocular disease. The eyes are kept straight by the drive to keep the image of the object being viewed in the centre of the macular area, where highest definition and colour vision is located. The tone in the extraocular muscles is constantly being readjusted to maintain this fixation. If the vision is impaired in one or both eyes this constant readjustment cannot occur and one eye may wander.

The squint is an important sign, as the cause of impaired vision may be eminently treatable, such as a cataract or a refractive error. It is especially important in a child because,

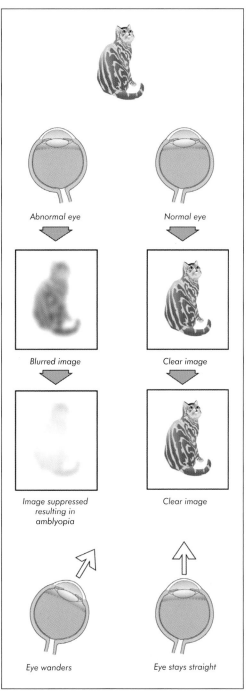

*Abnormal eye*          *Normal eye*

*Blurred image*          *Clear image*

*Image suppressed resulting in amblyopia*          *Clear image*

*Eye wanders*          *Eye stays straight*

A squint may be a sign of impaired visual acuity

---

**A squint is important**

- A squint may show that the acuity of the eye is impaired
- A squint may itself cause amblyopia in a child
- A squint may be a sign of a life threatening condition

---

unlike the vision of an adult, a child's vision may be irreversibly impaired if treatment is not given in time. The visual pathways in the brain that receive information from an abnormal eye fail to develop normally. The resulting depressed cortical function leads to amblyopia, commonly called a "lazy" eye. The child does not usually complain that the sight of one eye is poor. A pair of glasses to correct a refractive error may prevent a permanently impaired acuity.

**A squint may itself cause amblyopia in a child**. Misalignment of the eyes may be the primary problem, with resulting double vision. Young children do not normally complain of double vision. In a young child the vision of one eye may be suppressed to avoid this diplopia and the visual pathways then fail to develop properly. This leads to amblyopia of the eye that is otherwise organically sound.

**A squint may be a sign of a life threatening condition**. Squint is a common presentation in a child with a retinoblastoma. The resulting squint is non-paralytic and therefore the angle of deviation is the same, irrespective of the direction of gaze. The eye deviates because vision is impaired and this may occur in any eye with visual impairment.

A squint can also be caused by a sixth nerve palsy resulting from a tumour causing raised intracranial pressure. In this case the squint will be paralytic and the angle of squint will vary depending on the direction of gaze. Patients with myasthenia gravis may present with a squint and diplopia.

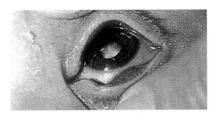
Congenital cataract

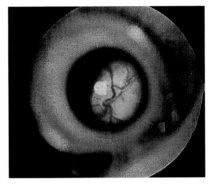
Retinoblastoma in a child presenting with a squint

## Clinical detection and assessment

Adults may complain of deviation of the eyes or of diplopia. For children, parents usually notice either one or both eyes turning in or out, or there may be a family history of squint. Children may also be referred from vision screening clinics.

### History

A family history of squint is a strong risk factor in the development of squint, and if there is any doubt the child should be referred. Children with disorders of the central nervous system such as cerebral palsy have a higher incidence of squint. Squint is more common in preterm infants. Problems during birth and retarded development also increase the likelihood of a squint. The parents' visual problems should be ascertained, particularly large refractive errors.

The earlier the age of onset, the more likely it is that an operation will be needed. A constant squint has a worse visual prognosis than one that is intermittent.

### Examination

*Check the visual acuity*

If the visual acuity does not correct with glasses or a pinhole, ocular disease or amblyopia must be suspected. This is particularly important in children, as the amblyopia or ocular problems must be treated immediately if sight is to be preserved. Visual acuity in infants is difficult to assess. A history from the parents is useful to find out whether the baby looks at them and at objects. However, if only one eye is affected the visual problem may not be apparent. If the sight is poor in only one eye, covering the good eye may make the child try to push the cover away.

*Look at the position of the patient's eyes*

Large squints will be obvious. Wide epicanthic folds may give the impression of a squint (pseudosquint), but children with wide epicanthic folds may still have true squints.

**Patients with myasthenia gravis may present with squint and diplopia**

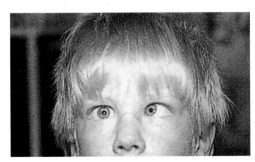
Left convergent squint: note position of light reflexes

**Infant vision testing is a time consuming procedure, but with patience it is possible to quantify the visual acuity even in young children by using matching techniques for pictures and optotypes (for example, LogMAR Kays picture matching cards)**

*Look at the corneal reflections of a bright light held in front of the eyes*
Note the position of the reflections; they should be
symmetrical. This test gives a rough estimate of the angle of any
deviation.

*Cover test*
Two types of cover test help to reveal a squint, especially if it is
small and the examiner is unsure about the position of the
corneal reflections.

- In the cover and uncover test, one eye is covered and the
  other eye is observed. If the uncovered eye moves to fix on
  the object there is a squint that is present all the time—a
  manifest squint. The test should then be carried out on the
  other eye. A problem arises when the vision in the squinting
  eye is reduced, and the eye may not be able to take up
  fixation. This emphasises the need to test the vision of any
  patient with squint. If the cover and uncover test is normal
  (indicating no manifest squint) the alternate cover test
  should be done.
- In the alternate cover test, the occluder is moved to and fro
  between the eyes. If the eye that has been uncovered moves,
  then there is a latent squint.

*Test eye movements in all directions of gaze*
If there is a paralytic squint, the degree of deviation will vary
with the direction of gaze. An adult will often say that the
separation of the images varies and that it increases in the
direction of action of the weakened muscles.

*Examination of the eye with a pupil dilating agent (mydriatic) and a
ciliary muscle relaxing agent (cycloplegic)*
Any overt abnormalities of the eye should be noted. Dilating
the pupil allows you to check for retinal disease, such as a
retinoblastoma, and the cycloplegic allows a check for any
refractive error. Adequate examination of the peripheral
fundus and refraction require dilation of the pupil and special
equipment. Cataracts and other opacities in the media, and the
white reflex suggestive of retinoblastoma, may be checked
without dilating the pupil, by observing the red reflex.

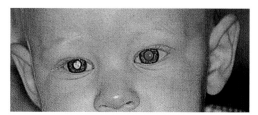
White reflex of retinoblastoma

# Management

## Paralytic squints

Paralytic squints usually occur in adults. Underlying conditions
such as raised intracranial pressure; compressive lesions; and
diseases such as diabetes, hypertension, myasthenia gravis, and
dysthyroid eye disease should be excluded.

If diplopia is a problem, one eye may need to be occluded
temporarily, for example, by a patch stuck to the patient's glasses.
Alternatively, temporary prisms may be stuck on to the glasses to
eliminate the diplopia. An operation on the ocular muscles may
be indicated if the squint stabilises. If an operation on the
muscles is either inappropriate or proves inadequate, permanent
prisms may be incorporated into the glasses' prescription.

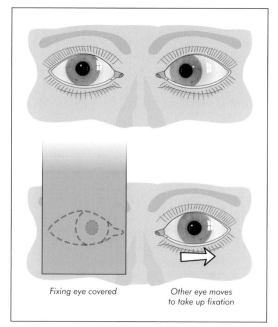
Fixing eye covered     Other eye moves
to take up fixation

Cover and uncover test

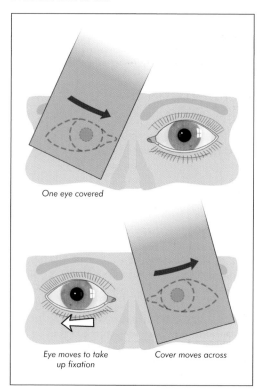
One eye covered

Eye moves to take     Cover moves across
up fixation

Alternate cover test

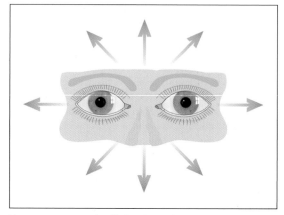
Test eye movements in all directions of gaze

Botulinum toxin is a recent addition to the diagnostic and therapeutic options in squint management. When injected into an extraocular muscle (under electromyographic control), the toxin produces a temporary reversible paralysis of the muscle. This technique can be used to alter extraocular muscle balance and correct squint, and it can be used to help predict the outcome of extraocular muscle squint surgery.

## Non-paralytic squints

Non-paralytic squints usually occur in children. If the squint is caused by disease in the eye that is causing reduced vision and subsequent deviation of the eye (for example, cataract) this needs to be treated. Treatments for non-paralytic squints are described below.

*Spectacles*

There are two main indications for prescribing glasses for children.

- A child who is hypermetropic (longsighted) and has a convergent squint. Normally when the ciliary muscle contracts the lens becomes more globular to allow the eye to focus on close objects (accommodation). This is linked to convergence so that both eyes can fix on the close object. If the child is hypermetropic the ciliary muscle has to contract strongly for the child to be able to focus on a near object. This excessive accommodation may cause overconvergence so that a squint occurs. This type of squint is called an accommodative convergent squint. The use of hypermetropic glasses in this case relaxes the ciliary muscles and removes the drive to overconverge.

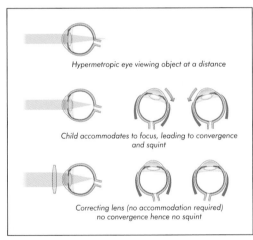

Use of spectacles to treat an accommodative convergent squint in a longsighted child

- A child who has a refractive error, particularly if this is unilateral. Because of the refractive error the image on the retina will be indistinct. The visual pathways will then not develop properly (resulting in amblyopia). Children with a refractive error may not develop a squint until the vision is poor in one eye, which emphasises the need to check the visual acuity. Glasses may prevent a child from developing severe visual loss in an otherwise "normal" eye—hence the need to refract every child with a squint or impaired vision.

*Occlusion*

This is the well known patching of one eye to encourage the development of the visual pathway of the "bad" eye. If the development of one pathway has been retarded by a squint or refractive error this pathway can be stimulated if the "good" eye

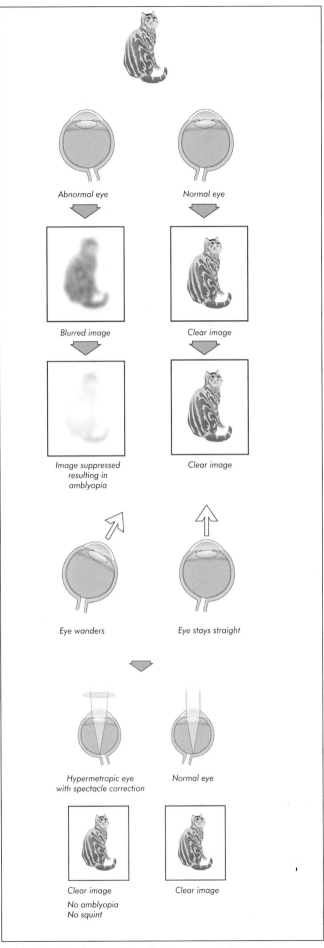

Amblyopia and squint caused by refractive error, and the use of spectacles to treat the refractive error and prevent amblyopia

is patched. However, this can only be done for a limited period, and there is a danger of the good eye itself becoming amblyopic. Most clinicians feel that after the age of about seven, occlusion therapy is unlikely to be helpful. In the meantime, the underlying problem must, of course, be corrected.

The vision of the good eye may also be "blurred" with drops such as atropine. Although there is much debate about the value of occlusion therapy, this therapy is useful for many children with specific types of amblyopia.

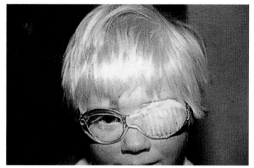

Occlusion of a child's good eye to stimulate the amblyopic eye

### Orthoptic treatment
A series of visual exercises may encourage the simultaneous use of both eyes.

### Surgery
The ocular muscles can be repositioned to straighten the eyes. Glasses are prescribed and occlusion performed before surgery, because an eye is more likely to stay straight if the vision is good. In adults "adjustable" surgery can be carried out. The muscle position is adjusted by altering the tension on the sutures postoperatively.

### Botulinum toxin
Very small amounts of botulinum toxin can be injected into overacting muscles to paralyse them for a few months. The treatment can then be repeated. It can also permit the assessment of the effect of prospective surgery before permanent surgery is carried out.

### In the older child
The effectiveness of treatment in reversing amblyopia decreases as the child gets older. Once the child is about 8 or 9 years old the visual system is no longer flexible and amblyopia cannot be reversed. However, the child may still need glasses to correct any refractive error, and an operation may be required if the squint poses a cosmetic problem.

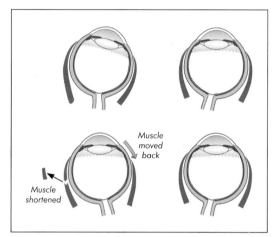

Operation for squint

# 12 General medical disorders and the eye

Most serious medical conditions affect the eye. It is important to know the ocular manifestations of systemic diseases for several reasons.

- *Screening can detect early ocular changes that may require treatment to prevent blindness.* A good example is a diabetic patient with new vessels on the optic disc, which signal an exceptionally high risk of visual loss unless treatment is given in time.
- *Knowledge of the ocular complications of other diseases may help in the diagnosis of an ocular problem.* A red, locally injected, and tender eye in a patient with rheumatoid arthritis suggests scleritis, which may progress to perforation of the eye. Iritis should be strongly considered in a young man with ankylosing spondylitis who presents with a red eye.
- *Ocular symptoms may suggest the systemic disease* (for example, prominent eyes and lid lag in hyperthyroidism) *or confirm it* (for example, the Kayser-Fleischer ring of copper in Wilson's disease).
- *Ocular signs may have prognostic value.* For example, if cottonwool spots occur in the eyes of an otherwise asymptomatic patient with AIDS, the prognosis may be poor.

## Diabetes mellitus

Diabetes mellitus is the most common cause of blindness among people of working age in the Western world. Two per cent of the diabetic population are blind, many of them in the younger age groups. Much of this eye disease can be treated, which makes early identification and referral crucial.

Cataract and primary open angle glaucoma are more common in diabetic than in non-diabetic patients. Cataract can be treated by surgical removal, and primary open angle glaucoma can be treated by drugs and operations that lower the intraocular pressure. Cataract can often be detected by viewing the red reflex; glaucoma by examining the optic disc. It is only too easy to forget to look for glaucomatous cupping of the disc when looking for signs of diabetic retinopathy.

Blinding diabetic retinopathy occurs in both insulin dependent and non-insulin dependent diabetic patients of all ages. For all categories of patient, the longer the duration of the diabetes, the more likely the patient is to have retinopathy (about 80% are affected after 20 years). However, the better the control of blood sugar levels, the lower the incidence of diabetic retinopathy. To avoid missing important signs, diabetic patients should have their fundi examined annually, by dilating the pupils with tropicamide 1%.

---

**Classification of diabetic retinopathy**

The current classification of diabetic retinopathy was introduced by the Early Treatment Diabetic Retinopathy Study (ETDRS):
- Non-proliferative diabetic retinopathy (NPDR) mild, moderate, and severe
- Proliferative diabetic retinopathy (PDR)
- Diabetic maculopathy

---

**Systemic diseases with ocular manifestations**

- Diabetes mellitus
- Hypertension
- Thyroid eye disease
- Rheumatoid arthritis
- Seronegative arthritides
- Giant cell arteritis
- Rosacea
- Sarcoid
- Behçet's syndrome
- Tuberculosis
- Congenital rubella
- AIDS

---

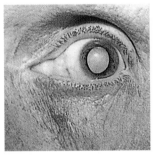

Cataract in a diabetic patient

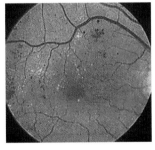

Background retinopathy: hard exudates, microaneurysms, and haemorrhages

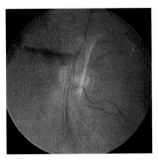

Proliferative retinopathy: new vessels, fibrosis, and haemorrhage

### Non-proliferative diabetic retinopathy

This is typified by microaneurysms, dot haemorrhages, and hard yellow exudates with well defined edges (called background diabetic retinopathy in some classifications). These changes do not have much effect on vision when they occur in the peripheral retina. However, there is a spectrum of changes in NPDR, some of which are associated with more ischaemic damage. These changes were previously classified as "pre-proliferative" retinopathy. The features of this more ischaemic moderate to severe NPDR are:

- Intraretinal microvascular abnormalities (IRMA)
- Cottonwool spots
- Deeper blotch and cluster haemorrhages
- Venous dilatation, beading and looping.

NPDR may coexist with diabetic maculopathy. The more ischaemic NPDR changes should alert the clinician to the possibility of progression to blinding proliferative diabetic retinopathy.

### Proliferative diabetic retinopathy

Typified by the growth of new vessels on the retina or into the vitreous cavity and thought to result from the ischaemic diabetic retina producing vasoproliferative factors that cause the growth of abnormal new vessels. These vessels may bleed, causing a sudden decrease in vision because of a vitreous haemorrhage. Worse still, this blood often results in the production of contractile membranes that gradually pull off the retina (tractional retinal detachment), causing blindness. This may occur in any diabetic patient, but more commonly is seen in young, insulin dependent patients. The vision may be 6/6 right up to the moment of a bleed, so early detection of new vessels by adequate fundal examination is crucial. Fluorescein angiography may help to identify areas of retinal ischaemia and new vessel formation. New vessels may also grow at the front of the eye on the iris and occlude the drainage angle of the anterior chamber causing glaucoma (rubeotic glaucoma).

Laser treatment (or any other method of photocoagulation) is used to treat proliferative retinopathy. The laser, however, is not usually used to coagulate new vessels as these may bleed or recur. When a patient has new vessels at the disc, the entire retina is treated with laser, except for the macula area, which preserves the central vision. This treatment, often called "panretinal photocoagulation" or "pattern bombing," destroys much of the ischaemic peripheral retina and stops it producing the vasoproliferative factors that induce the growth of new vessels, and often the new vessels regress. New blood vessels on the iris that block the outflow of aqueous and cause rubeotic glaucoma may also regress. However, thousands of laser burns and repeated treatments may be needed to achieve this. This treatment may substantially reduce peripheral vision and night vision and means that the patient may have to give up driving.

There is much current research in the development of clinically applicable antagonists to the vasoproliferative growth factors (for example, vascular endothelial growth factor (VEGF) antagonists).

### Diabetic maculopathy

Diabetic maculopathy may be divided into four types:

- Focal exudative macular oedema
- Diffuse exudative macular oedema
- Ischaemic maculopathy
- Mixed types.

When diabetic retinopathy causes vessel leakage and ischaemia in the macula area, central vision may be severely affected.

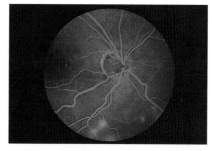

Fluorescein angiogram showing areas of leakage

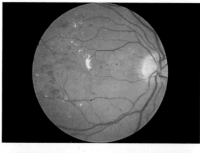

Non-proliferative diabetic retinopathy with macular changes and good vision: refer

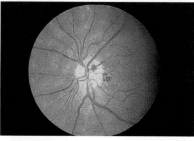

Proliferative retinopathy: refer immediately

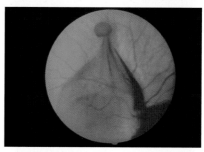

Diabetic vitreous haemorrhage

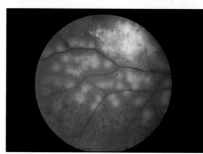

Diabetic retinopathy: recent and old laser burns

**Measures to improve prognosis in diabetic retinopathy**

- Control blood sugar
- Control hypertension
- Control hyperlipidaemia
- Stop smoking

Diabetic maculopathy is the major cause of blindness in maturity onset (Type 2) diabetes, but it also occurs in younger, insulin dependent diabetics. It may be amenable to focal laser photocoagulation, which may help to reduce any leakage, particularly when hard exudates are a prominent feature of the maculopathy.

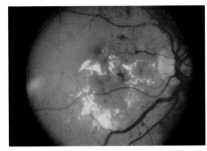

Diabetic maculopathy

### Screening for diabetic eye disease

Patients may be divided into five groups for screening purposes.

- Patients with no retinopathy or with minimal non-proliferative (background) retinopathy and normal vision when tested with glasses or pinhole. These patients can be reviewed yearly with dilation of the pupils. They should be told to attend sooner if there is a change in vision that is not corrected with glasses.
- Patients with non-proliferative (background) retinopathy and changes around the macula area. They should be referred to an ophthalmologist, as this may herald a blinding maculopathy.
- Patients with non-proliferative (background) retinopathy and impaired acuity not corrected with glasses or pinhole. The patient may have an oedematous or ischaemic form of maculopathy that is extremely hard to diagnose with the direct ophthalmoscope alone. The oedematous form may respond to focal laser treatment if this is given early.
- Patients with moderate to severe non-proliferative (preproliferative) retinopathy. They have no new vessels, but the haemorrhages are larger, the veins are tortuous, and there are cottonwool spots. These signs imply that the retina is ischaemic and that there is a high risk that new vessels will subsequently form. These patients should be referred.
- Patients with proliferative retinopathy. This is typified by new blood vessels, and sometimes cottonwool spots, fibrosis, and vitreous haemorrhages. These patients need immediate referral, particularly if there are vitreous haemorrhages.

In addition to ocular treatment, blood sugar should be carefully controlled. If the blood sugar concentration is brought under control rapidly, the fundus should be reviewed regularly during this period, as there may be a transient worsening of the retinopathy. There is no question that good control of the blood sugar level reduces diabetic retinopathy. Hypertension, renal failure, and hyperlipidaemia worsen the prognosis of retinopathy and must also be controlled. Patients should be strongly advised not to smoke.

Diabetic patients are also more prone to recurrent corneal abrasions, anteror uveitis, retinal vein occlusions, and cranial nerve palsies.

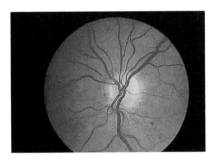

Non-proliferative diabetic retinopathy with good acuity: review regularly

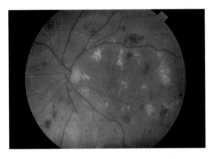

Non-proliferative diabetic retinopathy with reduced acuity: refer

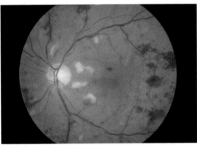

Severe non-proliferative diabetic retinopathy "Pre-proliferative": refer urgently

**Practical aids for diabetic patients with impaired vision include an audible click count syringe and a Hypotest instrument that gives an audible signal with urinary Diastix**

# Hypertension

The mild fundal changes of hypertension are extremely common. "Silver wiring" of the retinal arteries and arteriovenous nipping are well known signs, but arteriolar narrowing is the most reliable fundal sign.

Accelerated (malignant) hypertension is classically associated with swelling of the head of the optic nerve. Any patient with hard exudates, cottonwool spots, or haemorrhages as a result of hypertension has a grave prognosis. Patients with these fundal signs should have their blood pressure checked and diabetes excluded. Urgent referral to a physician is required as this combination of signs may not only result in blindness but is also life threatening. Retinal vein occlusion is also more common in hypertensive patients.

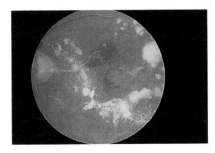

Retinopathy in accelerated hypertension with macular exudates and occluded vessels; disc swelling has resolved

# Thyroid eye disease

Patients may have signs associated with hyperthyroidism and the consequent overaction of the sympathetic system. These patients have retracted upper and lower lids caused by excessive stimulation of sympathetically innervated muscles in the eyelids. This also gives rise to the well known sign of lid lag when the patient looks downwards. These features may suggest the diagnosis when the patient walks into the surgery. If these signs are present, thyroid dysfunction should be excluded. If there are no visual problems, no corneal exposure, and the eyes move normally the patient need not be referred.

Patients may also have evidence of autoimmune disease directed against the orbital contents, particularly the muscles and orbital fat (thyroid autoantibodies may be positive). These signs may be associated with the classic signs of Graves' disease, including goitre, pseudoclubbing of the fingers (thyroid acropathy), hyperthyroidism, and pretibial myxoedema. Autoimmune orbital disease may also occur on its own with no thyroid dysfunction and with normal thyroid autoantibody status. The clinical features include the following, which may occur in any combination.

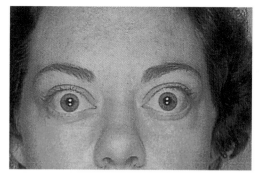

Hyperthyroidism with lid retraction

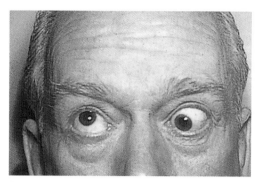

Autoimmune eye disease with restriction of ocular movements

- *Swelling of the eyelids*
- *Oedema (chemosis) and engorgement of the blood vessels of the conjunctiva*
- *Exposure of the cornea* because of lack of blinking and failure of the lids to cover the eye adequately
- *Pronounced protrusion (exophthalmos) of the eyes.* The absence of this feature in association with the other features may be even more serious, as a tight orbital septum may be holding back the swollen orbital contents. This may lead to a rise in intraocular pressure as well as pressure on the optic nerve
- *Restriction of eye movements.* This is caused by infiltration of the muscles with inflammatory cells, and consequent inflammation, oedema, and finally fibrosis. These changes can produce diplopia and strabismus
- *Optic neuropathy.* This is relatively rare. The fundal signs include vascular congestion and swelling or atrophy of the head of the optic nerve. There may be "folds" in the choroid caused by pressure on the globe. This should be excluded in any patient with autoimmune eye disease who experiences visual deterioration.

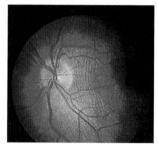

Choroidal folds

## Management of thyroid eye disease

- Associated thyroid dysfunction should be excluded, although treatment of any dysfunction may make no difference to the eye disease, and it may even make it worse
- Patients should be strongly advised to stop smoking
- Artificial tears and ointments should be used to lubricate the cornea and prevent drying and corneal ulceration (especially at night)
- If there are cosmetic or exposure problems caused by lid retraction, guanethidine 5% drops may reduce the lid retraction by relaxing the sympathetically controlled retractor muscles. Occasionally an operation on these muscles may be required
- If corneal exposure is threatening sight, the eyelids may have to be sewn together temporarily or permanently (tarsorrhaphy)
- Prisms incorporated in the patient's glasses may help to correct any double vision
- Operations on the muscles of eye movement may be required to realign the eyes in patients with longstanding diplopia that has stabilised. Recently, the introduction of local injections of

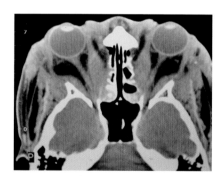

Radiology of thyroid eye disease

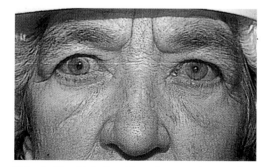

Patient with mild dysthyroid eye disease: red eyes and exposure as a result of infrequent blinking

minute doses of botulinum toxin to paralyse specific extraocular muscles has meant that patients with restrictive muscle diseases may sometimes be treated at an earlier stage
- In serious disease with corneal problems or pressure on the optic nerve, emergency treatment may be required, which may include high doses of steroids, surgical orbital compression, and radiotherapy. The visual fields may be restricted and there may be a relative afferent pupillary defect
- Changes in colour vision, which may be noticed while watching colour television, may be an important sign of optic nerve compression, and patients should be told to inform their doctor immediately if these changes are noticed

## Rheumatoid arthritis

Ocular complications frequently occur in rheumatoid arthritis. The lacrimal glands also are affected by an inflammatory process with consequent inadequate tear flow. The patient complains of dry, gritty, and sore eyes. Treatment consists of replacement artificial tear drops instilled as often as necessary. Simple ointment may also help, but this will blur the vision if used during the day. If there is an aggregation of mucus, mucolytic eye drops (for example, acetylcysteine) may help, but patients should be warned that these sting. In a few patients the "dry eye" syndrome may be sufficiently severe that there is associated corneal melting.

The inflammatory process may also affect the episcleral and scleral coats of the eye, causing the patient to complain of a red, uncomfortable eye. The redness is usually focal and there is tenderness over the area.

Scleritis is usually much more painful than episcleritis and the engorged vessels are deeper. If scleritis continues, the sclera may become thin (scleromalacia) and the eye may eventually perforate. The patient should be referred, as systemic immunosuppression may be indicated.

These processes may also occur in other connective tissue diseases such as systemic lupus erythematosus, scleroderma, and dermatomyositis.

## Seronegative arthritides

The seronegative arthritides include ankylosing spondylitis, Reiter's syndrome, psoriatic arthritis and arthritis associated with inflammatory bowel disease. Acute anterior uveitis (iritis, iridocyclitis) is much more common in these patients. If a patient with any of these conditions has a red eye, anterior uveitis should be suspected. This is particularly true if the patient has had past attacks, and "experienced" patients often know when an attack is coming on. The patient should be referred for early treatment, which may prevent some of the complications of anterior uveitis.

Seronegative childhood arthritis is a particularly important cause of chronic anterior uveitis. The great danger is that the eyes in this condition are often white and pain free, and the child may not complain of any visual problems. There may be secondary cataracts, which can cause irreversible amblyopia. Glaucoma secondary to the anterior uveitis may also occur and may be asymptomatic until the vision has been severely damaged.

The group of children particularly at risk are girls, those with fewer than five joints affected by the arthritis (pauciarticular), and those with antinuclear antibodies in

---

**In a patient with thyroid eye disease**
- Protect cornea (exposure and ulceration)
- Prevent damage to optic nerve (compression)

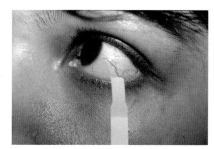

Dry eyes: Schirmer's test

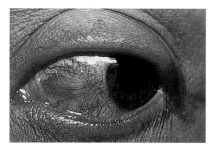

Episcleritis

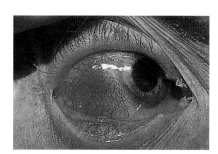

Scleritis

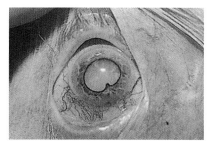

Chronic anterior uveitis and secondary cataract in seronegative arthritis

---

**Risk factors for ocular involvement in childhood seronegative arthritis**
- Female sex
- Fewer than five joints affected
- Antinuclear antibodies

their blood. These children should be referred to an ophthalmologist.

## Rosacea

Rosacea may seriously affect the eyes. There is often associated severe blepharitis, which may result in recurrent chalazia and styes. The abnormal lids and lipid secretion affect the tear film and "dry eye" symptoms result. The cornea scars, particularly in the inferonasal and inferotemporal areas, with neovascularisation. Thinning occurs and occasionally the cornea may perforate.

Treatment with tear substitutes is indicated together with treatment for any associated blepharitis. Systemic tetracycline (250 mg four times daily for up to a month, then daily for several months) may considerably improve the patient's ocular as well as facial condition (avoid using tetracycline in pregnant or lactating women).

## Sarcoid

Sarcoid is associated with various ocular problems. Acute uveitis and chronic uveitis occur, which may result in cataract, glaucoma, and a band of calcium deposited in the cornea (band keratopathy). The lacrimal glands may be infiltrated, resulting in "dry eye" symptoms that require tear replacement. The granulomatous process may affect the posterior part of the eye as vasculitis and sometimes infiltration of the optic nerve.

## Congenital rubella

The ocular manifestations of congenital rubella are extremely important. The child may have severe learning difficulties and be deaf, so early recognition of ocular problems and their treatment are vital. The eyes are often microphthalmic and associated treatable defects include cataract, glaucoma, squint, and refractive errors. The cataract may not appear until several weeks or months after birth, so the eyes should be re-examined. There may be a diffuse retinopathy ("salt and pepper" appearance).

## Acquired immune deficiency syndrome (AIDS)

The ocular complications of AIDS can be blinding and include retinitis, retinal detachment, papillitis, and cystoid macular oedema. Manifestations of ocular human immunodeficiency virus (HIV) infection include Kaposi's sarcoma of the conjunctiva and lids, HIV microvasculopathy (retinal haemorrhages and cottonwool spots), and vasculitis. Ocular cytomegalovirus (CMV) infection presents as a slowly progressive necrotising retinitis with areas of retinal opacification and haemorrhages and exudates along the vascular arcades. About 20-30% of patients with CMV retinitis will develop a retinal detachment.

Various antiviral agents have proved useful in the treatment of ocular complications, but they may have to be taken continuously, and systemic side effects from these treatments are common. The use of agents such as ganciclovir, foscarnet, cidofovir, and more recently fomivirsen has proved to be very effective in controlling CMV retinitis. Intraocular implants that release local antiviral agents reduce systemic complications.

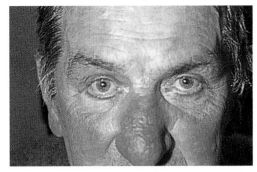

Rosacea and associated blepharitis

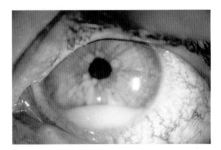

Hypopyon uveitis

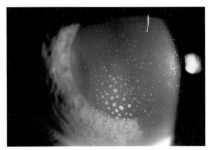

Keratic precipitates

---

**Ocular manifestations of congenital rubella**

- Cataract
- Squint
- Refractive error
- Glaucoma
- Retinopathy

---

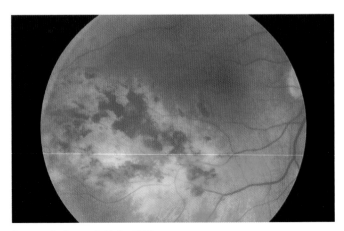

Cytomegalovirus retinitis in AIDS

Blindness resulting from the ocular complications of AIDS used to be one of the major reasons for suicide in AIDS patients.

The development of highly active antiretroviral therapy (HAART), with combinations of drugs including nucleoside reverse transcriptase inhibitors, non-nucleoside reverse transcriptase inhibitors, and protease inhibitors has dramatically reduced the incidence of ocular CMV infection.

Advances in therapy now result in improved immune function in many AIDS patients and new ophthalmic manifestations of AIDS are emerging. These include inflammation of the vitreous (vitritis) and accumulation of fluid at the macula (cystoid macular oedema).

# 13 The eye and the nervous system

## Nerves of eye movement

Ocular signs may be the first indication of serious neurological disease. Alternatively, the eyes may be responsible for "neurological" symptoms such as headache.

Palsies of the third, fourth, and sixth cranial nerves all cause paralytic squints, in which the angle of squint varies with the direction of gaze. Adult patients may also complain of double vision. It is important to exclude palsies of these three nerves when examining patients who have a squint, double vision, or both. In any patient with diplopia you should consider the possibility of ocular myasthenia gravis, which can mimic many different conditions.

### Third nerve palsy

Patients with a third nerve palsy may present with a variety of symptoms, depending on the cause of the palsy. These include a drooping eyelid, double vision (if the lid does not cover the eye), or headache in the distribution of the ophthalmic division of the trigeminal nerve.

On examination there is characteristically a ptosis (paralysed levator muscle of the eyelid) and the eye is turned out because of the action of the unaffected lateral rectus muscle that is supplied by the sixth nerve. The eye is sometimes turned slightly downwards because of the unopposed action of the unaffected superior oblique muscle supplied by the fourth nerve. The pupil is dilated if the parasympathetic fibres of the third nerve supplying the sphincter pupillae have been damaged.

Important causes of a third nerve palsy include intracranial aneurysms, compressive lesions in the cavernous sinus, diabetes mellitus, and trauma. If there is pain and a dilated pupil, a compressive lesion must be excluded urgently, as life saving curative treatment may be needed for what could be a fatal lesion, such as an aneurysm.

### Fourth nerve palsy

This is often difficult to diagnose. Patients may complain of a combination of vertical and torsional diplopia, which may be worse during activities such as walking down stairs or reading. There may be a compensatory head tilt, with the head tilted away from the side of the lesion and the chin depressed. The fourth nerve is long and therefore is particularly susceptible to injury. A patient with bilateral fourth nerve palsies following a head injury may complain only of difficulty in reading. This occurs as a result of difficulty during depression and convergence of the eyes because both superior oblique muscles are paralysed.

This diagnosis is easily missed if a careful history is not taken, and it should be considered in any patient who complains of difficulty in reading after a head injury.

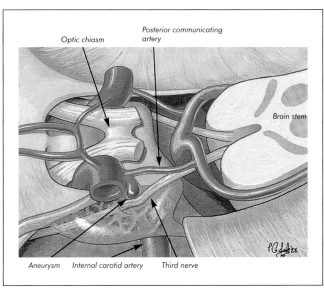

Posterior communicating artery aneurysm compressing third nerve

---

**Aetiologies of third nerve palsy**

- Aneurysm
- Microvascular occlusion
- Tumour
- Trauma

---

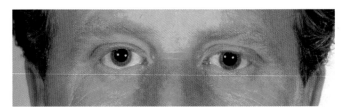

Fourth cranial nerve palsy—right hypertropia (see inferior scleral show) due to trauma. Signs are easily missed

---

**Aetiologies of fourth nerve palsy**

- Congenital
- Head trauma
- Microvascular (including diabetes and hypertension)
- Tumour
- Aneurysm

---

### Sixth nerve palsy

This is probably the best known of the palsies of the three nerves of ocular motility. The eye on the affected side cannot be abducted. The patient develops horizontal diplopia that worsens when they look towards the side of the affected muscle.

### Management of paralytic squint

A detailed ophthalmic, neurological, and general medical assessment is essential in order to make an accurate diagnosis. If diplopia is a problem, opaque sticky tape may be placed over the patient's glasses or a patch may be placed over the eye. Adults will not develop amblyopia. Temporary prisms can be put on the glasses if the angle is not too large. For long term treatment, permanent prisms (which are clearer than temporary prisms) may be incorporated into a prescription for glasses.

Later, an operation may be performed to straighten the eyes. Botulinum toxin may be injected into the extraocular muscles as a diagnostic or therapeutic procedure in paralytic squint.

> A sixth nerve palsy may be the result of raised intracranial pressure that is causing compression of the nerve

**Aetiologies of sixth nerve palsy**
- Tumour
- Microvascular occlusion
- Trauma
- Aneurysm
- Raised intracranial pressure

**Management of paralytic squint**
- Diagnosis
- Patch
- Temporary prism
- Permanent prism
- Botulinum toxin
- Operation

# Facial nerve palsy

### Seventh nerve palsy

Facial weakness caused by a seventh nerve palsy is common. In many cases no cause is found and the palsy improves spontaneously. If the eyelids do not close properly, corneal exposure, ulceration, and eventually scarring and blindness may occur. Ocular assessment should include the following.

*Testing of corneal sensation*
The cornea is innervated by the ophthalmic branch of the fifth nerve, which may also be affected by the pathology that is causing the seventh nerve palsy. If the corneal sensation is impaired, patients cannot feel foreign bodies or when their corneas are ulcerating. They should be referred to an ophthalmic surgeon, as there is a high risk of corneal scarring. When the seventh nerve is affected the patient is unable to close the eye and there is inadequate lubrication of the cornea.

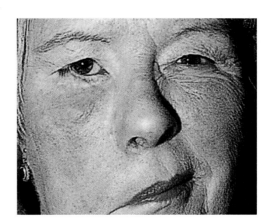
Right facial nerve palsy. The eyelids on the right have been partly sewn together to protect the eye

*Testing of Bell's phenomenon*
(Not to be confused with a Bell's palsy.) Normally when the eyes are closed the eyes move up under the upper lids. This "Bell's phenomenon" can be tested by observing the position of the cornea while the patient closes their eyes. If the cornea does not move up under the paralysed lid, the patient is at a high risk of developing corneal exposure.

*Staining the cornea with fluorescein*
Staining of the cornea when fluorescein is used indicates that the cornea is drying out. If there is only a tiny amount of stain, the eye is white and unremarkable on external examination, and the visual acuity is normal, the patient may be managed in the short term with tear drops and ointment. If the staining persists or if the eye becomes red then the patient should be referred immediately to an ophthalmologist. The cornea may need to be protected by frequent lubrication and by sewing together the lateral parts of the eyelids or lowering the upper eyelid with botulinum toxin.

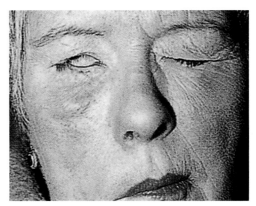
Cornea moves up under upper lid on attempted closure of the eye

## Sympathetic pathway

### Horner's syndrome

In a patient with Horner's syndrome the sympathetic nerve supply to the eye is disturbed. The clinical features are as follows.

- *A small pupil that is reactive to light* (unlike the small pupil caused by pilocarpine eye drops) because the sympathetically innervated dilator muscle of the pupil is paralysed.
- *A drooping eyelid.* The muscles that raise the eyelid are innervated by the third nerve and also by the sympathetic nerve supply. Therefore lesions of either the third nerve or the sympathetic nervous system supplying these muscles cause a ptosis, although in the latter case it is only slight.
- *Lack of sweating on the same side of the face* is because of sympathetic denervation and depends on the position of the lesion. The ocular movements are completely normal, as the extraocular muscles are not sympathetically innervated.

## Optic disc

### The swollen optic disc

There are many causes of a swollen optic disc, the best known of which is raised intracranial pressure resulting in the development of papilloedema. The absence of papilloedema, however, does not exclude raised intracranial pressure. The history and examination of the patient should lead to the suspicion of raised intracranial pressure, and a swollen optic disc is merely a helpful sign. The vision of patients with papilloedema usually is not affected until late in the course of the condition.

Most causes of a swollen disc are serious from either the ocular or systemic point of view, and patients should be referred promptly. If a patient has a swollen optic disc the following features suggest a diagnosis other than raised intracranial pressure.

### Impaired vision

Vision usually is impaired only late in the course of papilloedema. Impaired vision may indicate giant cell arteritis and the patient may or may not have aching muscles, malaise, headaches, tenderness over the temporal arteries, and claudication of the jaw muscles when eating. The disc is characteristically swollen and pale because the small vessels that supply the head of the optic nerve are inflamed and occluded. By this time vision will be severely affected. **It is important to exclude giant cell arteritis in any patient over 60 with visual disturbance or a swollen optic disc**, as urgent treatment with steroids is needed to prevent blindness in the other eye.

### Ocular management of seventh nerve palsy

The aim of treatment is to prevent corneal exposure and ulceration with subsequent complications of infection and perforation. Simple initial measures include frequent ocular lubrication with artificial tears and ointments and lid taping to physically close the eyelids. In more severe cases it may be necessary to reduce the size of the palpebral aperture surgically by performing a lateral tarsorrhaphy or by inserting an inert gold weight into the upper eyelid. Nerve reconstructive surgery can restore innervation to the facial muscles in severe cases.

**Ocular management of seventh nerve palsy**
- Frequent ocular lubrication (day and night)
- Eyelid taping to close lids
- Lateral tarsorrhaphy
- Gold weight insertion into upper lid
- Nerve reconstructive surgery

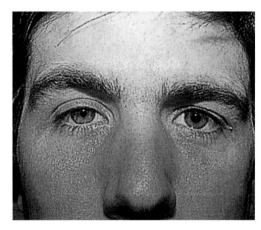
Horner's syndrome

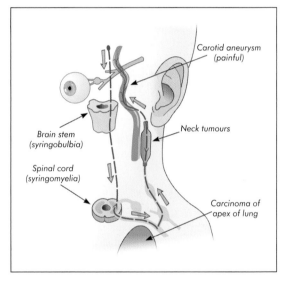
Sites of lesions of the sympathetic pathway to the eye

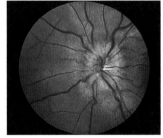
Papilloedema: swollen disc secondary to raised intracranial pressure

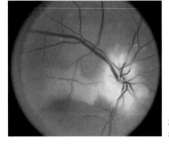
Swollen disc secondary to temporal arteritis

*Disturbance of the visual fields*

The visual fields of a patient with raised intracranial pressure usually are normal. A field defect usually indicates some other diagnosis, such as compression of the optic nerve.

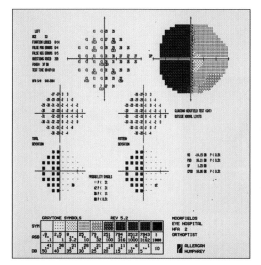

Visual field: bitemporal hemianopia caused by pituitary adenoma

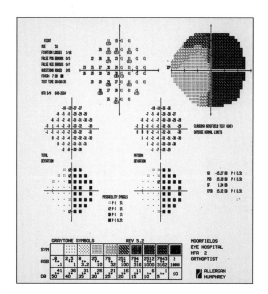

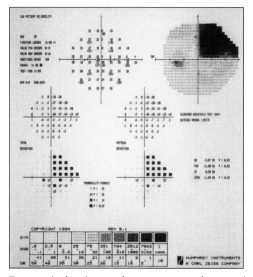

Computerised perimetry—homonymous quadrantanopia due to a stroke

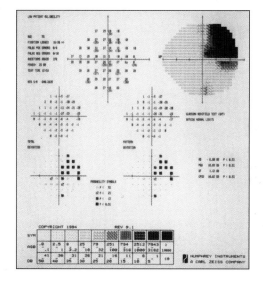

*A pale disc*

The disc of a patient with raised intracranial pressure is often hyperaemic. It is only in longstanding papilloedema that the disc becomes atrophic and pale. The disc is also pale if the swelling results from ischaemia of the optic nerve, as in giant cell arteritis.

*Retinal exudates and haemorrhages*

These are present in papilloedema and are usually found around the disc. If there are many exudates or haemorrhages in the retina, diagnoses such as retinal vein occlusion, malignant hypertension, diabetes, and vasculitis should be considered. In all patients the blood pressure should be measured and the urine tested for the presence of sugar, blood, and protein.

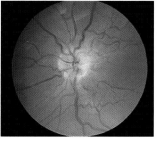

Optic neuritis

*Conditions that may mimic swelling of the optic disc*

- *Longsightedness* (hypermetropia), in which the margin of the optic disc does not look clear. A clue lies in the patient's glasses, which make the patient's eyes look larger.
- *Drusen of the head of the optic nerve*—These colloid bodies of the head of the nerve makes the margin of the disc look blurred.
- *Developmental abnormalities of the head of the nerve*—These may be difficult to diagnose.

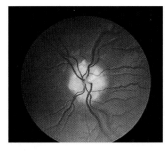

Optic nerve head drusen

## Management
Patients with true papilloedema will need neurological investigation. Patients with pseudopapilloedema and other acquired causes of optic disc swelling (for example, retinal venous occlusion, uveitis, optic neuritis, ischaemic optic neuropathy, optic nerve compression, and optic nerve tumours) will need full ophthalmic and neurological examination and investigation.

## The pale optic disc
There are many causes of a pale optic disc and it is vital to make the correct diagnosis, as many of them are treatable. These include compressive lesions, glaucoma, vitamin deficiency, the presence of toxic substances (for example, lead or some drugs), and infective conditions such as syphilis. It is also important to identify whether the cause is hereditary, as genetic counselling, and occasionally, metabolic treatments are available (for example, a diet free of phytanic acid and plasma exchange may prevent the progression of ocular disease in Refsum's disease).

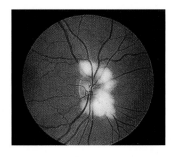

Myelinated nerve fibres

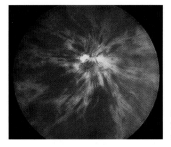

Swollen disc secondary to central retinal vein occlusion

# Headaches and the eye

Most patients who present with a history of "headache" around the eye do not have serious disease. The following features in the history and examination should raise suspicion of serious disease.

- *The nature of the headache*—Headaches that cause sleep disturbance or that are worse on waking or with coughing, suggest raised intracranial pressure. Temporal tenderness in patients over the age of 60 with symptoms of aching muscles and malaise suggest giant cell arteritis.
- *Visual disturbance*—If there is a change in visual acuity that cannot be corrected by a pinhole test, serious disease should be suspected. A history of haloes around lights (caused by transient oedema of the cornea when the intraocular pressure rises) suggests attacks of angle closure glaucoma.
- *A red eye*—In acute glaucoma the eye is usually red, injected, and tender, and the acuity is diminished. The pain is deep seated and may be associated with vomiting. Inflammation of the iris and ciliary body also cause a red eye and a deep pain. Primary open angle glaucoma does not present with severe pain.
- *Defective ocular movements*—Restricted ocular movements on the same side as the pain may indicate serious disease, including orbital cellulitis (from infected sinuses), inflammatory lesions in the orbit, and compressive lesions causing nerve palsies (for example, a posterior communicating aneurysm causing third nerve palsy and pain around the eye).

---

**Aetiologies of the swollen optic disc**

**Pseudopapilloedema**
- Optic disc drusen
- Hypermetropia
- Congenital anomaly of hyaloid system

**Papilloedema**
- Blockage of ventricular system
- Blockage of cerebrospinal fluid absorption
- Dural venous sinus thrombosis
- Space occupying lesion
- Hypersecretion by choroid plexus tumour
- Idiopathic (benign) intracranial hypertension

**Acquired swelling of the disc**
- Eye disease—Retinal vein occlusion or uveitis
- Vascular—Hypertension or ischaemic optic neuropathy
- Inflammation—Optic neuritis
- Drug related—Ethambutol, isoniazid, or streptomycin
- Infiltrative—Sarcoid, lymphoma, or leukaemia
- Metabolic—Thyroid eye disease
- Compression—Optic nerve glioma or meningioma
- Disc tumour—Glioma or haemangioma, or metastatic

---

**"Headache" around the eye: important features**
- Nature of pain
- Associated visual disturbance
- Red eye
- Defective ocular movements
- Abnormal pupils
- Abnormal optic disc

---

- *Abnormal pupils*—An abnormal pupil on the side of the headache should suggest a compressive lesion (for example, a painful Horner's syndrome caused by an internal carotid artery aneurysm). Pupillary abnormalities and ocular motility problems may be present in so called "cluster headaches" and "ophthalmoplegic migraine," although these are relatively benign conditions. However, patients with headache around the eye, together with ocular motility or pupillary abnormalities, should be investigated to exclude serious lesions.

- *Swelling, atrophy, or cupping of the optic disc*—A patient with headaches around the eye in addition to any of these symptoms should be referred. The swelling and atrophy may be due to a compressive lesion and pathological cupping suggests a chronic form of glaucoma.

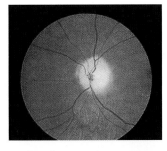

Optic atrophy

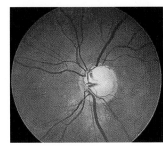

Glaucomatous cupping

# 14  Global impact of eye disease

## Impact of blindness worldwide

**Every five seconds an adult goes blind somewhere in the world, and every 60 seconds a child goes blind.** Using the World Health Organization (WHO) definition of blindness, defined as vision in the better eye of less than 3/60, it is estimated that there are about 45 million blind people in the world. There are also about 135 million people who are visually impaired and who need help.

## Leading causes of blindness worldwide

Ninety per cent of the world's blind and visually impaired people live in the countries of the developing world. The impact of medical progress has been greatest in the more affluent countries of the developed world, where economic resources have facilitated significant advances in tackling blinding diseases.

Two hundred years ago the main cause of blindness in western Europe was smallpox; 100 years ago this was replaced by ophthalmia neonatorum. Although there are success stories in the battle against blindness, it is important to remember that blinding diseases still represent one of the major problems facing developing nations.

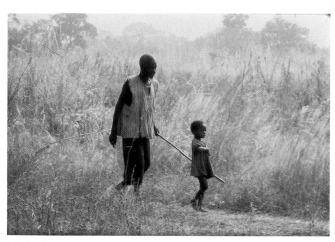

Whole villages are affected by river blindness caused by *Onchocerca volvulus*. Photograph reproduced with permission from the Christian Blind Mission

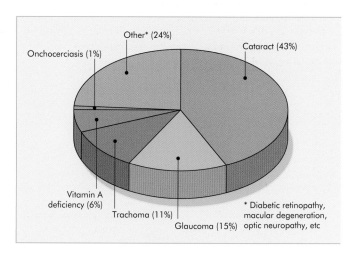

Pie chart of causes of world blindness

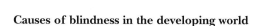

**Main causes of blindness in the developing world today**

- Cataract
- Glaucoma
- Trachoma
- Vitamin A deficiency
- Onchocerciasis

**Causes of blindness in the developing world**

*Cataract*

About 20 million people are blind in both eyes because of cataracts. These people could all be treated if they had access to cataract surgery, and currently there are large scale programmes under way in many developing countries.

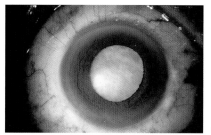

Cataract

*Glaucoma*

If glaucoma is detected at an early stage then blindness is usually avoidable. However, long term topical glaucoma therapy is not practicable in many low income countries, because of cost, compliance, and access issues. Currently several research programmes are evaluating the feasibility of surgery. In areas of the world where angle closure glaucoma has a high prevalence, laser therapy (peripheral iridotomy) has the potential to prevent much blinding disease.

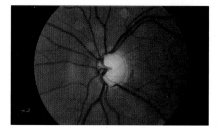

Glaucoma—cupped disc

## Trachoma

Infection with *Chlamydia trachomatis* causes this severe scarring conjunctival infection. Basic hygiene and public health measures can dramatically reduce the prevalence of blinding infection.

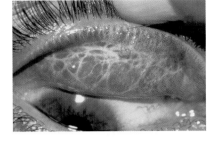

Severe trachomatous scarring of tarsal conjunctiva

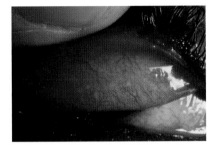

Conjunctival infection with *Chlamydia trachomatis*

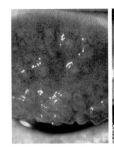

Chronic inflammation of tarsal conjunctiva secondary to chlamydial infection

## Vitamin A deficiency

Vitamin A is needed to maintain epithelial surfaces (including the ocular surface) and to make retinal photoreceptor pigments. Deficiency of vitamin A (xerophthalmia) causes ocular surface dryness, scarring, infection with possible perforation, and night blindness. Vitamin A supplementation can eradicate this important blinding disease, which, coupled with common childhood infections (such as measles), is a major cause of blindness in children.

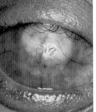

Corneal scarring caused by vitamin A deficiency

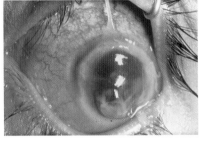

Corneal melt after measles in vitamin A deficient patient

## Onchocerciasis

"River blindness" is caused by the parasite *Onchocerca volvulus*, carried by the blackfly, which transfers the parasite when it bites humans. Infection results in corneal scarring, cataract, glaucoma, and chorioretinitis. Treatment with ivermectin can help control parasite levels in infected individuals, and public health measures to eradicate the blackfly vector, which breeds in fast flowing rivers, can reduce disease prevalence.

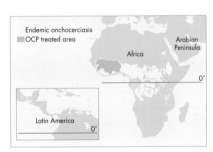

Areas affected by onchocerciasis

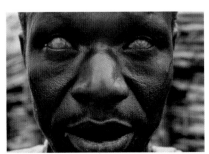

Corneal scarring caused by onchocerciasis

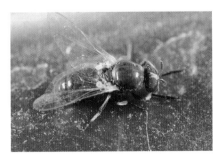

Onchocerciasis—blackfly vector

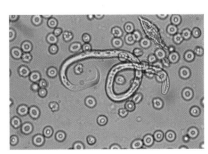

Onchocerciasis—parasite

### Main causes of blindness in developed countries

- Age-related macular degeneration (ARMD)
- Glaucoma
- Cataract
- Diabetic retinopathy
- Refractive error

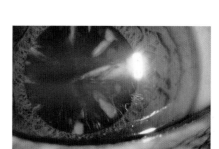

Age-related macular degeneration

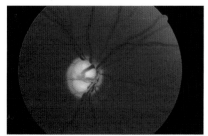

Glaucomatous cupping of optic disc

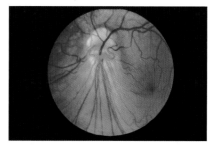

Cataract

## Changing nature of blindness in "middle income" countries

Many South American and eastern European countries now fall into this economic category. The extreme poverty common in the developing world is not so prevalent in these countries, and there are pockets of very high quality ophthalmic care. Two ophthalmic diseases in particular have the potential to increase dramatically in prevalence in "middle income" countries: retinopathy of prematurity and diabetic retinopathy.

### Retinopathy of prematurity (ROP)

The prevalence of blinding ROP is increasing in many "middle income" countries because basic neonatal intensive care facilities are available. Although better neonatal care means more babies survive, there are usually very limited facilities for monitoring babies. As a result, many babies receive unmonitored supplemental oxygen therapy and therefore are at increased risk of developing severe ROP.

### Diabetic retinopathy

As the levels of income, nutrition, and basic health care increase, more patients with type 1 and type 2 diabetes will survive into later life. Many of these patients will develop sight threatening diabetic retinopathy, but there is simply not enough access to laser treatment facilities to manage their retinopathy and prevent blinding complications.

"Dragged" optic disc and macula due to peripheral scarring and contraction of retina

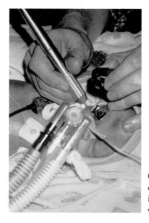

Cryotherapy for treatment of retinopathy of prematurity being performed in intensive care while baby continues to be ventilated

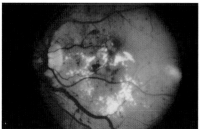

Diabetic maculopathy

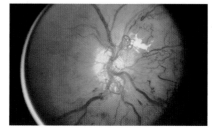

New vessels on optic disc in proliferative diabetic retinopathy

# Eye disease in patients from outside the United Kingdom

With modern air travel, the number of people travelling to the United Kingdom from developing countries has increased dramatically. An overseas patient with an ophthalmic problem may have a tropical ophthalmic disease not usually seen in the United Kingdom (for example, red eye due to trachoma) or an ophthalmic manifestation of a systemic disease (for example, red eye and uveitis secondary to tuberculosis).

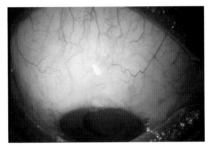

Granulomatous uveitis—for example in tuberculosis

# Travelling outside the United Kingdom

Many patients will ask their family doctor for ophthalmic advice before travelling. Some common questions are answered below.

### Can I fly after surgery for retinal detachment?

Patients who have had gas injected inside their eyes to provide tamponade as part of surgery for retinal detachment should consult their ophthalmic surgeon before flying, as it usually takes several weeks for the potentially expansile gas (sulphur hexafluoride) to be absorbed postoperatively. Aircraft cabins are usually pressurised (to about 8000 feet) during flight, which can cause the intraocular gas to expand while the plane is in the air, leading to acute glaucoma.

### How soon after eye surgery can I go abroad?

All patients who have had intraocular surgery (for example, cataract surgery) are at risk of delayed complications such as inflammation or infection for the first two to four weeks post operatively. The patient should consult their ophthalmic surgeon before arranging travel abroad.

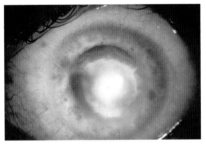

Postoperative glaucoma drainage bleb

### Should I take any precautions because of my eye problems?

- Patients who are prone to recurrent uveitis or corneal herpetic disease may experience a reactivation of their problem while abroad. Patients should carry basic information about their condition with them and may carry a supply of appropriate medication in case of a flare up. It is always best to seek an expert ophthalmic opinion before starting therapy abroad
- Patients who have had previous glaucoma surgery may benefit from carrying a supply of topical antibiotics in case they develop an infective conjunctivitis
- Individuals that wear contact lenses should pay strict attention to hygiene when using lenses in developing countries. Non-sterile water (for example, from taps) used to clean contact lenses or contact lens cases may be a source of pathogens such as acanthamoeba, which can cause intractable, potentially blinding infection. Care should be taken with contact lens hygiene, especially if wearing contact lenses on long haul flights. Daily wear contact lenses should not be worn overnight on long flights, because the cabin partial pressure of oxygen is reduced considerably
- Patients with "dry eye" syndromes may experience a marked exacerbation of their symptoms in the dry atmosphere of the aircraft cabin and should carry a supply of ocular lubricants.

Contact lens related corneal abscess

It is estimated that over the next two decades the number of blind and visually impaired people in the world will double to 360 million

# Summary

The global population is **increasing** and **ageing** rapidly. As population demographics change, the prevalence of sight threatening disease will also change. Global initiatives, such as **Vision 2020: "the right to sight,"** which aim to eliminate avoidable blindness by 2020, set us all a daunting challenge.

# Index

Please note that page references in **bold** refer to figures and those in *italics* refer to tables/boxed material.

# Index

# Index

# Index